a coauthor book led by Deirdre Slattery

FITNESS TO FREEDOM

create inner peace and self confidence
by breaking unhealthy cycles

a coauthor book led by Deirdre Slattery

FITNESS TO FREEDOM

create inner peace and self confidence
by breaking unhealthy cycles

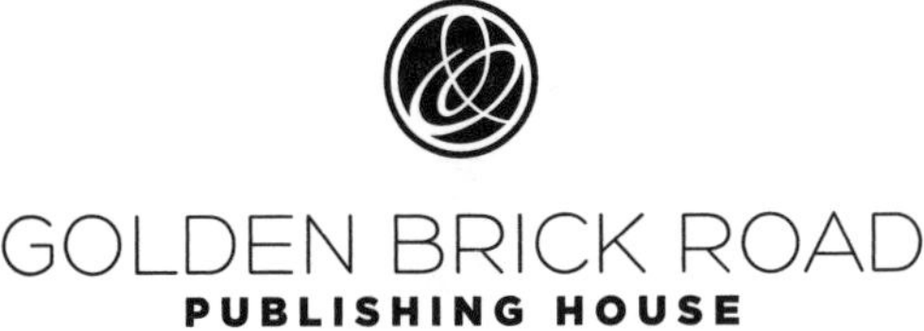

2019 Golden Brick Road Publishing House Inc. Trade Paperback Edition

Published in Canada, for Global Distribution by Golden Brick Road Publishing House Inc.

www.goldenbrickroad.pub
For more information email: kylee@gbrph.ca

ISBN:
Paperback: 978-1-988736-73-0 **kindle:** 978-1-988736-83-9
ebook: 978-1-988736-82-2

To order additional copies of this book: orders@gbrph.ca

TABLE OF CONTENTS

INTRODUCTION

BY: DEIRDRE SLATTERY

Fitness to Freedom has come to mean many things to the women who've played a role in this book and for countless others who have become connected through building this project. Fitness can come and go in our lives, serving different purposes in different seasons; its many forms are beautiful and offer so much, not only physically but on a deep level within, connecting and grounding us emotionally and spiritually. Whatever your fitness sanctuary — the gym, hiking trails, soccer fields, or your own living room — this space truly supports you in a practice of peace and harmony. Our hope is that, just like your favorite fitness space, this book can provide support and encouragement on your journey from fitness to freedom as you seek balance, peace, and harmony in your life.

My personal fitness story started with a simple desire to step up my life using the tool I knew and loved: purpose-driven exercise. Although this decision started with me, for myself, it ultimately blossomed into a larger story, with more and more people helping each other to live their best lives and reach their goals.

The recognition of your potential and ability can come from having to overcome a difficult time and simply trying to survive. It may come while you're trying to meet a specific goal or benchmark. However it happens, this miraculous ability to see your own power can transform you and inspire you to live to your fullest potential. When you see your worthiness and your power to live strong, healthy, and free, you begin raising your standards and seeking a better quality of life. Listen to that inner voice saying that you can do more and that you deserve more. The more I listen to that voice, the more I am able to do, the more grateful I become, and the more I am free to give back to others. This is the magic and the secret behind bettering your life — desiring to improve, watching the spark ignite, feeling more satisfaction, bringing in opportunity and possibility, and sharing this new fire and light with others.

When I began using fitness to lift my life from the ground up, I also found a renewed inner strength and self-confidence. I built muscles not only in body but also in mind so I could begin to better manage what life has to offer. Through this journey, I have gained more tools and allies to help me live a life with more meaning, depth, and purpose than I ever could have planned or dreamed was possible.

What does living free mean to you? Twenty-one women have come together in this book to share the meaning they've developed through their unique life experiences, their struggles, and their achievements. This is powerful, real talk from accomplished fitness leaders, powerhouses, and amazing women who simply wish for more from life. These warriors may appear to be living lives that are out of reach, but in these chapters, they all share simple truths behind their success. Our goal in this book is to break down the barriers around seemingly impossible goals so that they become not only plausible but achievable, doable, and relatable. We hope our stories give you the confidence to do all that you are dreaming of, and all that you have yet to dream into existence, as well as to find more peace and love for yourself. We also hope to inspire more women to come together, lift and empower one another, and give space to be heard, feel safe, and be unapologetically ourselves.

Some of us have taken on fitness late in life, while others have moved through different forms of exercise before finding their best fit. If you have ever wondered what is like to take fitness to the next level and brave the world of competition, we also share many unique views into this part of the industry — the good, the bad, and the ugly. Despite our different experiences, there are common themes running through all our stories. Many of us have been told that we are too much or not enough. We have felt doubt, have backed down from our dreams due to fear, and have done things because we believed we had to fit in, until we broke the mold and made our own design.

This book will acknowledge that life is difficult. Motivation and inspiration don't always feel present, and failure and discouragement are a part of the journey. But you have the power within you to live with purpose and drive, to take care of yourself, and to serve others.

There is no one path to follow in this book, no right or wrong way to read it; it's simply a collection that you can pick up at any page or chapter. Take from it what you need that day or that moment. Respecting and loving yourself at any stage in life can be a challenge, but learning to be at peace with yourself at all stages is the ultimate goal. We are all moving our bodies and minds throughout the day, and it's up to us to choose how. The women brought together to make this book have all experimented with the best way to honor their bodies with exercise, food, and mind work. Each one of us has a different recipe that best meets our needs and gives us flow, peace, and balance in our lives. You need to decide on the safest and healthiest way for you. A physical gym is not the only place to train our bodies and minds; in fact, the gym can be everywhere and anywhere you choose. We encourage you to see through our varied stories that there are countless ways to live your best life!

No matter what your health and fitness goals are, your "why" will be the best clue to how to create and adopt your fitness regime. You are stronger than your excuses, and you are worthy of feeling your best. Here's to the start of your next chapter in health, fitness, and life and to reaching beyond what you have known and experienced before. Here's to living free in body, mind, and spirit.

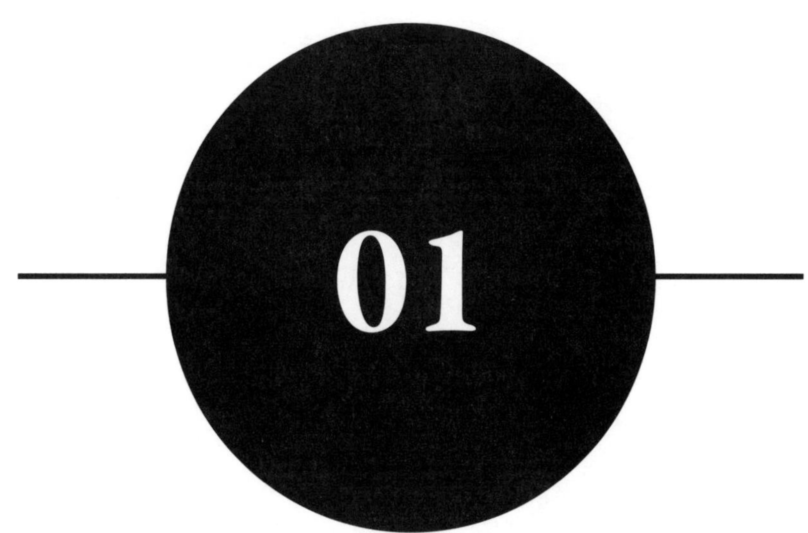

THE FREEDOM TO ACHIEVE

01

I CAN

"Our minds are extremely compliant. They carry out what we instruct and accept what we think and say as truth."

BY: ALLISON MARSCHEAN

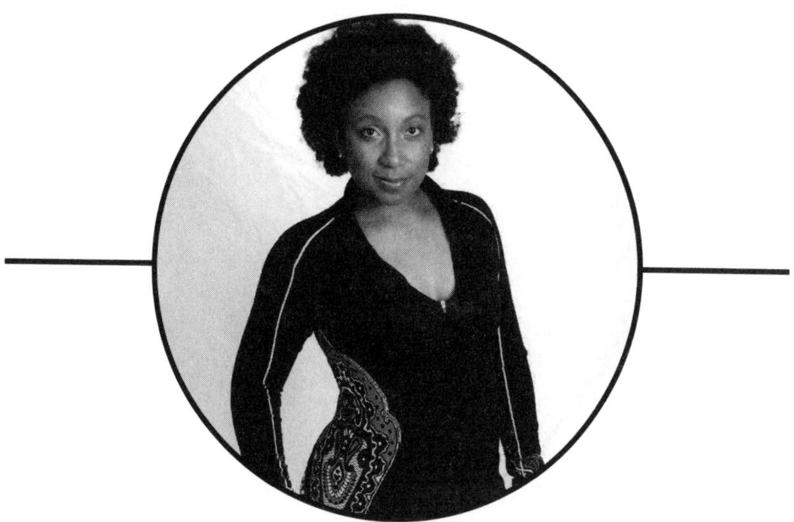

Allison's parents instilled in her the importance of "I can" thinking, and over the years, she's had numerous opportunities to apply that lesson. She's excited to share the power that accompanies a mind set on success.

Allison and her husband Vince have three daughters — eight-year-olds Brynn and Piper and two-year-old Jordan. Allison majored in French at The United States Military Academy at West Point, NY and graduated in 2001 with a bachelor of science in systems engineering. She also holds a master of science in management of technology from Murray State University and a master of arts in organizational psychology from Columbia University's Teachers College. Allison is a flat-vending fundraiser. She sells stickers and temporary tattoos to raise funds for non-profit organizations, and has served as an officer in the United States Army and Army Reserves for eighteen years.

www.allisonmarschean.com

fb: @allison.marschean | ig: @allison_marschean

li: allison-marschean-b22988108

You *can* do it!!

Maybe you've heard this a thousand times and maybe you haven't. Either way, guess what? You get to hear it here! The one thought I want you to take away and believe in fully by the end of this chapter is, "Yes! Yes, I can!" All the stories you've been told or are telling yourself that include the words "I can't" — throw them out now!

Did you know that our minds believe what we instruct them to believe? The mind is extremely compliant. It carries out what we instruct and accepts what we think and say as true, even about ourselves. The words we speak and think have the power to either propel us to greatness or hold us back.[1]

Let's say that for a good portion of your formative years, you were told you are uncoordinated and terrible at sports. You've heard the story so often that it has worked its way into your subconscious. Eventually, this becomes the story you tell yourself. For example, even though cycling doesn't take much coordination, you turn down an opportunity to join your friends in a bikeathon because "you are uncoordinated and terrible at sports." This psychological phenomenon is known as a self-fulfilling prophecy; it is what happens when a person's belief influences their behavior in a way that eventually shapes their reality. Essentially, it is a belief that comes true because we think and act as though it is already true.

The term self-fulfilling prophecy, also known as the Pygmalion Effect, was coined in 1948 by sociologist Robert K. Merton; while this effect can play out negatively, it can also work in our favor.[2] When someone's belief about themselves is positive in nature, they tend to experience positive outcomes. Professor Henry Higgins and Eliza Doolittle from the 1964 film *My Fair Lady* are terrific examples of how self-fulfilling prophecies play out. *Eliza* wants to replace her unintelligible Cockney accent with something more refined so she can work in a florist shop; Higgins, a noted phonetician, believes he can remedy her problem. Ultimately, they talk themselves into accomplishing their goals.

---

[1] Allen, James. (2011). *As a Man Thinketh.* USA: Best Success Books.

[2] Crossman, Ashley. (2019, March). Definition of Self-Fulfilling Prophecy in Sociology: The Theory and Research Behind the Common Term. Retrieved from https://www.thoughtco.com/self-fulfilling-prophecy-3026577.

As the Bible says, "[t]he tongue has the power of life and death, and those who love it will eat its fruit."[3] If you tell yourself that you are capable of reaching a fitness level beyond your current abilities, then you are likely to do the work to make it happen, thereby reinforcing your new belief.

LET'S GO BACK

I was fortunate to be born to parents who always told me I could achieve anything I set my mind to. They taught me the importance of doing my best and discouraged me from comparing myself and my performance to others. I learned that measuring myself against others was not only unproductive, it was also self-limiting. Spending time pining over how we rate in comparison to someone else is a total energy suck. Evaluating our performance for the sake of self-improvement, however, is both practical and reasonable.

Initially, I applied my parents' instruction primarily to academics. I recall getting frustrated by the fact that I struggled with some subjects that came so easily to other students. Eventually, I came to understand that I needed to spend my energy on learning the material, not on trying to figure out why some other kid understood the concept the first time around. This lesson eventually carried over to other areas of my life and paid dividends.

While I didn't completely stop trying to figure out why some people performed better than I did in some areas, I did redirect my efforts toward strengthening my own abilities. I tried to keep 1 Corinthians 10:31 in mind: "[s]o, whether you eat or drink, or whatever you do, do all to the glory of God." This meant that I needed to perform to the best of my ability, even when my best was not better than someone else's.

Perhaps you're thinking, "I wasn't as fortunate as Allison; my parents were nothing like hers. They never encouraged me or saw more in me than I saw in myself." You can't alter your past, but you can choose how to move forward with your goal now. There is always

[3] Proverbs 18:21 NIV.

a way to move beyond those things that do not serve us; there are always opportunities to begin believing that you can.

KEY PRINCIPLES

Know Your Goal.

When I applied to West Point, one of the application questions asked why I wanted to attend The Military Academy. I listed four reasons, and one of them was to stay in shape — you can't help but stay in shape when you join the military! The U.S. Army does a terrific job providing Soldiers with the standards they need to perform well. Times, repetitions, weights, and scores are all spelled out. There is no guessing what it takes to succeed, and there's no excuse for failing. The first fitness test I had to pass to gain admission to West Point was the Physical Aptitude Examination (PAE) . The PAE is a multi-event fitness test that all Candidates must pass to continue with the admissions process. When I received the scoring table, I decided to strive for the top score in every category. My combined score was 582 which was well above the minimum requirement. Always go in knowing your goals and what you need to do to achieve them. Showing up with the ability to achieve the goal you set should be a non-negotiable.

Six years after I took the PAE, I found myself setting another significant goal. I was a Second Lieutenant by then and was determined to earn the Gold German Proficiency Badge. Several events were involved in this challenge, including a swim, a sprint, a weapons proficiency test, and the big one — the thirty-kilometer road march, to be completed in three and a half hours while carrying a twenty-five pound rucksack. I trained for the gold, and the gold is what I earned! I did that thirty-kilometer march in the Arizona heat and beat several of the men on the course. When I passed one guy, he asked if I was on the first loop and was shocked when I told him I was on the second. After I passed him, I set my sights on each person I saw and made it my goal to catch up and pass them as well.

As long as you know the standard and practice the events, you can!

There Will be Setbacks. Do Not be Discouraged.

Your limitations in the present moment are not permanent, or at least many of them aren't. We tend to use anything we view as a limitation in our lives as an excuse not to move forward. Those limitations can range from our socioeconomic status to a sprained ankle to an itchy case of poison ivy or even something more severe, like the loss of a limb or our eyesight. But all these factors can shift. Socioeconomic status can change for the better. A sprained ankle will heal. The incessant itch of poison ivy eventually fades, and even the limitations associated with the loss of a limb or eyesight can be overcome and worked around. We *will* encounter speed bumps in life. As such, it's imperative to recognize that we have a choice. We can view setbacks as either permanent or temporary.

Over the years, I've experienced physical injuries that temporarily prevented me from accomplishing significant milestones in my military career. I arrived at the 101st Airborne Division at Fort Campbell, Kentucky in late 2001 to serve as an Intelligence Officer in the 716th Military Police Battalion. As a healthy and fit new Second Lieutenant assigned to this historic and noteworthy division (think *Band of Brothers*), I was acutely aware of the requirement for every officer to be Air Assault-qualified and to proudly wear the coveted Air Assault badge on their uniform.

In an effort to ensure that units send only their best to the Sabalauski Air Assault school, the Army requires candidates to complete a challenging obstacle course and a rigorous twelve-mile road march with full military gear in under three hours. I trained for these challenges and proved that I was fully capable of attending the school. Unfortunately, between the date I completed the road march and the date the course began, I strained muscles around my hip and was not able to attend the course. Since the pre-qualification test has a shelf-life, it expired before I was fit to start school. This scenario happened again and again. I eventually completed the twelve-mile road march and the obstacle course three times before I ever went to Air Assault school! You can probably imagine how tiresome this was, but as discouraging as setbacks can be, we must keep our end state in mind, reminding ourselves how badly we want it.

Know Your Limits.

To enjoy freedom through fitness, it is also imperative to know your body and its limits at any given point in time. I've spent eighteen years in the United States Army, ten on active duty and eight in the Army Reserves. In the Army, a stigma surrounds people who are injured, like a black cloud following them around. When a Soldier sustains an injury or is ill, he or she goes to the doctor who then writes a medical excuse form called a profile. This places limitations on physical activity. Soldiers who repeatedly receive profiles become known as "Profile Rangers" or "Profile Riders", and all good Soldiers know that "Profile Riders" are weak. At least that's the stigma. Of course, Soldiers do legitimately require a physical profile from time to time, but people who abuse the profile system make difficult for those with real needs. In fact, some people who really should have a medical excusal refuse to get one to avoid the stigma associated with them.

In 2006, I was playing in my last soccer game at Fort Huachuca, Arizona before heading to Fort Lee, Virginia. During the game, I took a spill going for the ball; I left the emergency room later that night with a half cast and crutches. My left foot was destroyed. What was my new command going to think of their new staff officer?

I showed up to my new unit with a profile and one soft orthopedic Velcro shoe. It was embarrassing. You never want to show up to new unit with an injury or a profile. It makes for a poor first impression. I'll never forget when I first met with the Deputy Commander. He asked me, "So, how'd ya hurt your foot?" When I answered, "Soccer," he gave a short laugh and said, "Soccer? Okay," as if he found it hard to believe.

Several months, numerous doctor appointments, and one fall off a folding chair later, I learned that I'd sustained a Lisfranc injury: all of the ligaments that held my midfoot together were torn. By April 2007, I was fully recovered and worked up to running the two-mile physical fitness test again. It wasn't my fastest time, but given the circumstances, I did rather well. For most of my time in the unit up to that point, I hadn't been able to run, so most people in the unit had no idea what I was capable of. At the end of that two-mile run, a female Soldier said, "Ma'am! I didn't know you could run!"

Injuries and setbacks suck. However, you must get past yourself and your ego and allow your body to heal. Remember that your body will be with you longer than your present circumstances. You've got to take care of yourself.

Be Your Greatest Competition.

"Each one should test their own actions. Then they can take pride in themselves alone, without comparing themselves to someone else, for each one should carry their own load." - Galatians 6:4-5 NIV

In 2013, someone saw me in my Army uniform in the library and invited me to meet her trainer to see about joining his fitness competition team. In her opinion, he wouldn't have to do much to get me ready to compete. While I was flattered, I tucked the idea away for over a year. By summer 2015, the timing was right and finances were available, so I connected with the trainer and got to work. During the month of August, I was traveling so I practiced at-home workouts. In September and October, I worked with the trainer once a week and worked out on my own the other days of the week to get ready for a November competition. I didn't have much time to prepare; however, I'd made up my mind to do the work required to be stage-ready.

I wasn't in it to win. Believe it or not, the thought of standing on a stage in a bikini did not thrill me — I don't even wear bikinis. I was in it because someone saw something in me that I'd never considered, and I wanted to go for it. I simply set out to do my personal best. When competition time came around, there were definitely women who had less body fat than me and women who had been training longer, but given the short timeline, I was proud of what I accomplished. An added bonus was taking second place in the Military Division! I've found that when our modus operandi is to see how we measure up to others, our subconscious minds dwell on that comparison even when we're not actively sizing up those around us. I could not have done my best if I had been focused on comparing myself with the other competitors.

POWERFUL POINTS TO REMEMBER

Optimism Can Be Learned: The Origins of an Optimistic Mindset.

Martin E. P. Seligman, Ph.D., defines our outlook on life and our habitual explanation for events as an explanatory style; unlike portions of our intelligence and other psychological traits, these explanatory styles are learned, not inherited.[4] We learn optimism and pessimism as children from our primary caretakers. In general terms, whatever a primary caretaker's explanatory style is, the child will develop a similar style. The good news is that the explanatory styles developed in childhood can be overridden and replaced with new habits that promote optimism.

Visualization Works!

I receive periodic emails from motivational speaker and "cheerleader of dreams" Terri Savelle Foy. In the midst of writing this chapter, I received an email entitled *Visualizing Will Change Your Destiny.* While I don't know what my destiny is, I have experienced the power of visualization in my own life. My parents introduced me to visualization. On more than one occasion, they had me close my eyes and see myself successfully accomplishing the task at hand. For instance, when there was a gymnastics move I was struggling with or was just afraid to try, I'd close my eyes and watch myself doing it perfectly. I played it like a tape on a loop in my head over and over. I applied this same exercise to pitching in softball, taking tests in school, and even applying for highly sought-after assignments in the military. Try it for yourself. Repeatedly see yourself accomplishing your goal in your mind's eye and experience the power that follows.

You can do it! Yes! Yes, you can!

---

[4] Seligman, M. E. P., PhD (2006). *Learned Optimism: How to cChange Your Mind and Your Life.* New York, NY: Vintage Books.

02

LOST AND FOUND

*"Conformity keeps us safe and trapped.
A free and happy life begins by first noticing what it is we truly desire and then being grateful for every step on the journey to achieving it."*

BY: BARB SOTOS

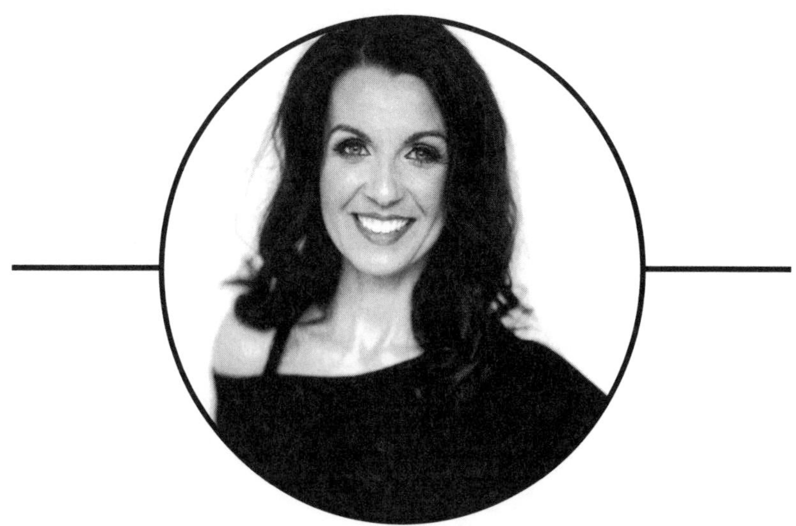

Barb Sotos is passionate about helping people cultivate awareness and gratitude in order to live a life more aligned with their desires. This passion led her to become a yoga teacher. Barb holds a bachelor of science from the University of Western Ontario and has completed yoga teacher training, along with certifications in restorative yoga, yoga with weights, and indoor cycling. Barb is a gratitude coach and is working toward a holistic weight loss expert certification. She developed and ran an empowerment camp for girls and also leads workshops on identifying personal desires and creating a vision for a life incorporating those desires. She teaches yoga at corporate locations and at various gyms and studios, as well as at the Regional Rehab Centre to individuals with newly acquired brain injuries.

Barb makes people feel safe when they need to express their feelings, and she has a talent for bringing a calm positivity into a space. Her clients have described her as "a teacher who has a wonderful ability to mix the physical challenge of each practice with a thoughtful dose of mindfulness. She seems to have the intuitive ability to know precisely when you need to calm your thoughts and not let your mind race away during any part of your practice."

www.barbsotos.com

ig: @livinyoga

I always felt like I was different. Born to immigrant parents and living between two countries, I never fully integrated into one way of life or the other. I felt like a true misfit. While my upbringing allowed me to see early on that there are many different ways to live life, this view was unlike that held by those around me. This created an isolating inability to relate. I quickly learned that the best way to fit in and be accepted was to silence my voice.

As a teenager, I struggled with my weight, gaining and losing fifteen to twenty pounds yearly. In my early twenties, my mother lost her two-year battle to cancer. While my peers were just starting their lives, with new careers and independence and dating, my world came to a crashing halt. I found myself yet again in a situation to which those around me could not relate. Depression and isolation set in, and I lost a drastic amount of weight. My desire to disappear was manifesting through my body, yet the world saw something different. I received so many compliments for my weight loss, which made me feel even more isolated. My digestive issues got worse, but if I tried to talk to my friends about not feeling well, their response was, "You're fine, you can afford to eat whatever you want, you're skinny!" When I got pregnant, I gained over seventy-five pounds and I struggled to lose that weight. I tried and failed at almost every diet out there, unable to sustain any of them. I felt down about myself. By this point, I had only a few people in my life, mostly by choice to protect myself from the pain of more loss. I was hitting an all-time low.

It was during this part of my life that I stumbled upon the practice of yoga and the journey of cultivating awareness and gratitude. These practices helped me peel back the layers and barriers I had put up that were not serving me well. I started to uncover and identify who I was and what I was passionate about. I realized the power in becoming vulnerable and going deep into self-reflection to identify where I had created patterns and mechanisms to keep myself safe and how my own views kept me isolated in my self-created prison.

Have you ever experienced a sudden moment of awareness and thought, "How did I get here?" In that moment, were you flushed with a rush of panic? You might have felt disconnected, or maybe like you were standing alone in the realization that not only did you never plan to be in this place but that you also have no plan for where to go from here. Perhaps an anxious and urgent feeling kicked in at the thought that a good portion of your life had passed without you being present to experience most of it. The good news is, you can decide how you want to live the rest of your life and be present for it every step of the way from here on out. The key is the awareness.

Awareness brings the life back into life. It allows us to become co-creators of the life we desire by identifying our passions, seeing what we want our life to look like, and then taking action to make it happen. Cultivating awareness is difficult work and takes ongoing effort. It involves identifying areas in ourselves that may be painful to approach: beliefs that are limiting, fears we have developed, and behavioral patterns acquired in response to those fears. When you take a vulnerable approach to determining who you are and what you want out of life, you can then take small steps to change those patterns and to make choices that align with your desires. Being vulnerable means facing difficult truths, stepping out of the familiar, adding or removing relationships, and starting to take responsibility for your choices. Awareness of the self brings back control over the relationships you keep, the job or hobbies you hold, the exercise you perform, and the food you eat. So if you find yourself thinking, "Things never work out for me", or "I am not that lucky," you can start to change these patterns through awareness.

Change is terrifying, but it is the only constant in life. We need to truly embrace change and learn how to actively flow through it. As Lao Tzu said, "[l]ife is a series of natural and spontaneous changes. Don't resist them; that only creates sorrow. Let reality be reality. Let things flow naturally forward in whatever way they like."[1] This is how I started my change, and it is how I help my clients start theirs.

First, I encourage you to write down the major areas of your life. These could include relationships, health, money, hobbies/interests, spirituality, and community. List one area per page so you have room to write. Under each heading, list how you presently feel about that area of your life.

Second, write what your heart craves to feel under each area. The key here is to write out what you desire, not what you think others would view as acceptable. Be true to you.

[1] Meah, A. (2019, January). 33 Inspiring Lao Tzu Quotes. Retrieved from https://www.awakenthegreatnesswithin.com/33-inspiring-lao-tzu-quotes/

Third, write down all the things you already do, and anything more you need to do, to feel the way you want to feel in that area of life.

Fourth, write down any obstacles and excuses that may impede you from doing those things. This part is the most overwhelming and, in my opinion, the area where we need to be the most empathetic, patient, and forgiving with ourselves. Soliciting help may be of great value at this stage, whether it's from a friend or a professional.

Finally, write down solutions to remove, lessen, or eliminate those obstacles or excuses. This could include setting stronger boundaries or asking for help. In *The Happiness Advantage,* Shawn Achor talks about lowering our barriers so that we can take the path of least resistance to reach the desired behavior. In this step, self-reflection and vulnerability play a crucial role. Start to pay attention to your thoughts, your triggers, and your patterns. Consider questions like:

- What emotions am I experiencing when I pay attention? Examples might include anger, shame, insecurity, fear, or depression.
- How does that emotion feel and where in my body do I feel it?
- Where do I fall into the same patterns? Examples might include venting, eating, shopping or humiliating others.

Acknowledging our patterns is an important part of the journey to awareness. Here are examples of what this exercise might look like.

First: I feel fatigued, stressed, and negative toward myself.

Second: My heart craves to feel vital, feminine, graceful, strong, flexible, and balanced.

Third: To achieve my desired feelings in this area, I could do yoga, indoor cycling, meditation, or strength training. I could make more nourishing meals even when I am rushed, eat more vegetables, drink more water, eat less chocolate, be consistent with my gratitude journal, and keep my self-talk positive.

Fourth: When I am in a rush, I choose junk food; my excuses include I don't have time, I feel tired, or I have nothing in the house to make a quick and nourishing snack. To clear out those obstacles, I will carve out time during the week, play some music I enjoy, have containers ready for meal prep, and cut up food items to quickly throw together when needed.

I also don't have many people in my inner circle. The ones I do have don't share my passions, my views, or my goals. I will look for a networking group that I can join to make relationships that will help inspire and support my desires.

Fifth: I will set timers to limit my social media surfing. These timers can also serve to remind me to check in with my thoughts, see how I may have avoided or reacted to situations, and start to identify my patterns. Then I will break down the steps into smaller blocks. I want to feel vitality, which I can achieve by eating more nourishing meals, which means I will grocery shop and meal prep, which means I will need ideas and containers. One measurable step I can take today is looking for some recipes, writing out a grocery list, or pulling the containers out of my cupboard.

The steps to change don't have to be big and overwhelming; you just have to take action toward change. I picked up a great tip from Mel Robbins' audiobook, *Take Control of Your Life*. She suggests that you focus on your goal, not on the things that stand between you and that goal. For example, if you want a bagel, you can either look at the line at the store and think about the time it will take for you to wait or you can look at the bagel itself and then the line is no longer an obstacle. Consider how you want to feel and what you need to do to feel that way, identify your obstacles, excuses, or fears, and figure out how you will reduce or eliminate them. Once you have identified how you want to feel in each area of your life, we move into the next stage: visualizing yourself living your desired life.

I see myself starting my day doing yoga, and that vision makes me feel strong, flexible, and graceful. I see myself drinking lemon water before and after my practice, and that makes me feel hydrated. I see myself engaging with others and having positive conversations after my yoga classes; that makes me feel connected. I see myself sitting to meditate and watch my thoughts once I get home, and then I see myself making and eating a nourishing meal. These things make me feel vitality and balance.

When going through this exercise during a workshop, I like to end by having my clients create a vision board with words, quotes, and pictures that evoke how they want to feel. I suggest you create such a board and keep it where you can see it daily. You can also edit anything that changes or no longer aligns with your passions.

This last exercise is life-changing and, in my opinion, the most important: keeping a gratitude journal. You can use an existing journal or shop for a new journal that makes you feel good. Take a few moments every day to write out three things you are grateful for. You could write down anything you happen to think about or you could have a schedule so that every day focuses on a specific area of your life. Next, write out why you are grateful for each of those things, followed by how it makes you feel to have those things in your life already. End the journal entry by expressing appreciation for your life.

For years, I felt disconnected from my body; no diets worked for me and exercise did not help. I also lived from a place of fear. I feared the pain of loss; I lacked faith and believed I had no control over my destiny. Although I was a positive person on the surface, my inner dialogue focused on what I felt was lacking. That thinking gave my control away to external sources.

Shifting my outlook and developing awareness of my thoughts and behavioral patterns and their direct effect on my choices had a massive impact on my life. Through awareness and gratitude, I started to train my mind to look for and focus on the things I have in my life, to make choices that make me happy, to see opportunities as they present themselves, and to decide whether they align with my desires. Awareness and gratitude have helped me listen to my body, eat nourishing foods that make me feel good, and not restrict myself to a limiting diet. I now choose activities that make my body and mind feel strong, feminine, and graceful. The cultivation of awareness of my inner life has changed my outer world. As Albert Einstein said, "[t]he world as we have created it is a process of our thinking. It cannot be changed without changing our thinking."[2]

---

[2] Five quotes from Albert Einstein about personal development. (2018, July 4). Exploring Your Mind. Retrieved from https://exploringyourmind.com/5-quotes-by-albert-einstein-about-personal-growth/

03

WHEN THE BEST IS NOT ENOUGH

"You are enough and perfect exactly as you are — don't let anybody tell you the opposite."

BY: VIOLAINE PIGEON

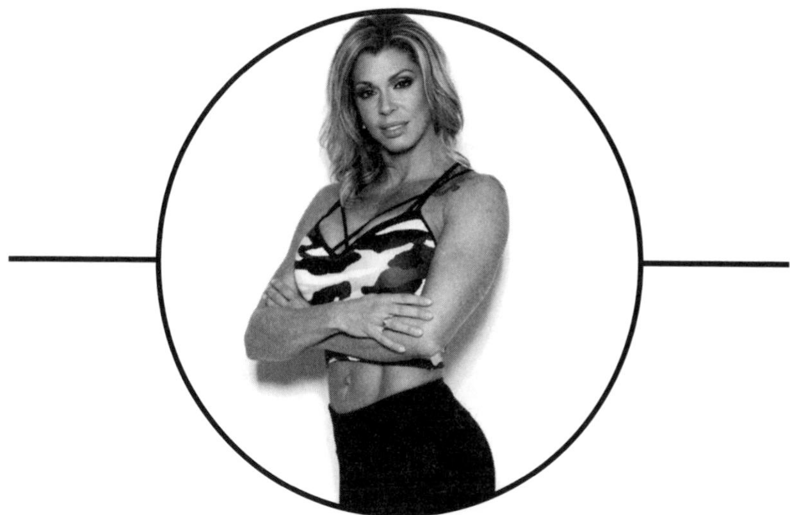

After studying at the University of Montreal as a dietician, Violaine started a clinician career in a larger hospital in Quebec. There she learned how to positively influence others to reach their health goals, as well as how to interact with her peers to become a real teammate in support of patients' well-being. Her personal experiences further strengthened her wish to become a healthy living role model, a positive example, and a balanced person for her family and for the rest of the world. She always wants to reflect the things she teaches.

Over the years, Violaine has become a motivating nutritionist and a wellness creator. She sees the good in every situation and aims to transmit that vision to her clients. She believes that humans can reach all they can dream of. Violaine is also an invested fitness athlete, a mother of two magnificent, happy small humans, Olivier and Chloé, and an overexcited wife-to-be to her fiancé Vincent.

Violaine lives close to Montreal with her family. She speaks French but has always read in English. This opportunity to write in an English book completed part of her bucket list. She believes this book is a wonderful way to reach the soul of a person and give them wings.

"You can do what you have to do, and sometimes, you can do it even better than you think you can" - Jimmy Carter

I am a perfectionist. For as long as I can remember, I have worked hard to meet my own expectations and feel satisfied about myself — in school, ballet classes, personal projects, social relations, and my career. All my life, I found it hard to accept that I was allowed to not be perfect.

But here is the question I have learned to ask: Am I a perfectionist because I want to be proud of myself, or did someone else tell me I *should be* perfect?

Only after facing some major hardships as an adult did I realize that I have typically focused on how other people perceive me. Before 2009, I did not understand that my perfectionism stemmed from my need to be told that I was good enough. I only saw the value in myself through the eyes of others: through their compliments, their comments, their perceptions. I also depreciated myself according to their judgments. While I thought I was doing things for myself, to satisfy myself, I was in fact just looking for approval from those around me.

Here is my story.

In October 2009, I had just gone back to work after my second maternity leave. Prior to going on leave, I had worked as a pharmaceutical sales field manager trainer for my province. Since my return, however, my company had promoted me to national medical affairs partner. I felt excited at first: new tasks, new manager, new opportunities to develop myself, and new people to meet. However, I was also a bit afraid of the end of my daily on-the-road role, as well as my new responsibility to travel for at least one week per month. Most frightening of all, for the first time, I had to work full-time in English. In other words, the new position presented a big challenge for me, as I speak French and I had a family life with very young kids. But I accepted the challenge.

A few months passed. The job was difficult every day; I tried to figure out how to execute my tasks to the best of my ability, but I was still struggling. I faced an even bigger issue in my relationship with my immediate supervisor. She lived in another province of the country, in another time zone, and we only had a virtual relationship. I have always loved to develop relationships with people, so I found it hard to work this way. Furthermore, I realized after a few months that this manager didn't work well with me. She made political comments about the fact that I came from the only francophone province of the country, as well as many bad comments about my teammates. Projects tasked to me would be cancelled after I had spent days or weeks working on them. I was uncomfortable, and that feeling only grew as time went on.

The final straw came in August 2010. It was time for my annual evaluation so I had to meet my manager in person. As we only met a few times before, I felt a little shy. The evaluation was crazy; it demolished me. I was a perfectionist and high-achiever, so it was a real trauma to be criticized for the fact that I had taken maternity leave twice, for the time I took to accomplish my tasks in another language (even though I was working evenings and weekends), and for the fact that I still talked to my previous colleagues and manager. There were no positive comments, no constructive criticisms, no appreciation for the things I had done well. I did everything to hold back my tears. I felt worthless. It broke me. When I went home, I was paralyzed. My heart, my soul, and my body all felt locked.

I was unrecognizable for months after that horrific meeting. In addition, my husband and I were struggling terribly and were in the midst of a divorce procedure. We were selling our dream house, I had to move to a small apartment and adjust to seeing my kids only part time due to shared custody, and I lost friends and familiar landmarks. All of these factors led me to a major breakdown. I isolated myself from everything and everybody, and I wasn't able to take care of the bare minimum for my family or for myself.

My doctor put me on work leave and introduced medications to balance my state of mind. This was hard to accept because I was judging myself. I saw myself as a loser, a failure. I could feel supportive for someone else affected by depression, but not for myself. It took time to recognize that I had tried too hard to fit in a box I prescribed for myself, I had completely forgotten about who I was. After a few weeks, I finally started to follow the medical prescriptions because I realized there was nothing else to do; I was unable to continue the road I had been traveling.

Time passed. After a few weeks of trying to heal and put my pieces back together, my insurance company contacted me to propose a new plan: the integration of physical activity as an additional support against the depression. Even though I used to be a very sociable and interactive person, I was terribly shy when it came to entering a gym and taking care of myself. Regardless of my fear, I complied with the recommendation and hired a personal trainer to break the wheel that held me prisoner. For the first time in my life, I asked for help. It was one of the best decisions of my entire life.

I started with two training sessions per week, always with my personal trainer to fight my shyness about working out. After the first month, I asked to increase our sessions to three per week. We had the opportunity to talk during my workouts, and it started to make me feel better. Then I gained the courage to work out without a trainer. It was my first victory in months, and I felt so happy. There was light at the end of the tunnel . . .

I followed this beat for months and started to be able to take care of my kids and myself properly. I revisited cooking (which was a very big win, as I'm a nutritionist), reading, and going out to see friends. I also noticed that I looked forward to every training session. After many weeks of reflection, I made some other major changes in the way I lived. I left my job and started to work as a private dietician. I also reorganized my schedule to integrate my workouts every week. I decided I deserved a better life, that I was worth it.

After two years, I had built an entirely new life, a new me! I dedicated myself to my new lifestyle. In my new role as a self-employed dietician, I helped people prevent and recover from health issues. Using workout plans from my trainer, I exercised alone four to five times a week. I had my smile, my self-esteem, my belief in *me* back. I was physically and mentally stronger than before all these dark episodes.

In fall 2011, I met another trainer in my gym. He told me he had noticed how hard I had worked for months and what a great improvement he saw in my shape and in my mind — I always looked dedicated to my plan and focused on my training. He was an athlete trainer and introduced me to competitive fitness. I felt excited by what he was presenting me, but I was also confused. Here I was, thirty-six years old, and all he was showing me were young athletes. I didn't feel like an athlete; I was simply a mother training to recover and stay in good health, body and soul. But he convinced me to try a real athlete lifestyle, and we set the goal for me to experience a fitness competition in six months.

In April 2013, for the first time ever, I jumped on a fitness stage. I brought back the bronze medal. In 2019, I will compete for the fifteenth time, at forty-three years old.

I discovered the satisfaction of reaching my goals through my fitness journey: not by the trophies and medals I won but through the determination, dedication, and focus I put in. I feel stronger than ever before in my life, both physically and mentally. I have also forgiven myself for what I first saw as weakness when I began this journey. Now I focus on the progress I've made instead of on what I missed. I have learned to establish and to be satisfied by my own criteria. I am living for myself and most of all, I now know that nothing is impossible.

One of the best lessons to learn in life is how to master who you are.

I'm not saying that you need to live the life of a fitness competitor to discover your inner potential. Rather, I'm saying that you need to find your own way to build your inner strength. Body, mind, and soul are related; one never comes without the other. If you become stronger physically, chances are you will become stronger mentally, too.

In the gym, we often say that the body can achieve what the mind believes. And it is true: if you look at a weight or an exercise regimen and doubt yourself and your ability, you program your mind to consider failure as an option. On the other hand, if you look at the same exercise and use your self-talk to say you will do it no matter what, your body will execute what you asked for. Thus, you can train your mind while you train your body.

There is always a way. Sometimes you can't figure it out at first sight, but with time, you will start to see different angles to a solution. Sometimes in the gym, we do not know how to execute a movement that requires a specific strength. We have to integrate new exercises to develop the muscles involved. When we do this, after a short time, we can perform what we first saw as impossible.

My advice: Stop trying to fit in a box designed by other people. Stop being afraid to take care of yourself before taking care of others. You have your own life, with your own experiences, values, and desires and your own strengths, qualities, and capabilities. It is your duty to explore them and to use them. They are your power and they are unique to you. Nobody else can fit in your shoes as you walk your life. Trying to make everyone happy often means not being happy yourself because you aren't listening to your own needs. To just fit in with the wishes of someone else often means to forget who you truly are. You deserve to be the first person considered in your own life. You need to try to make yourself happier, and the people who love you, the people who care about you, will be happy to see you blossom.

I learned something very important through the fitness world. I discovered that women are happy for the success of their sisters, that they cheer at other women's accomplishments, and that they value one another, regardless of their own background. Even if we meet in the context of a competition, we all make the effort to be there for one another. Everyone deserves to win. This is all we consider.

As long as your life is not over, it is not too late. I have received many comments saying that I am too old to embrace this fitness lifestyle. I have realized that those who were the most skeptical about my lifestyle were those with the most fear and the most excuses. They are not really judging my choices; they are afraid they are not able to do the same things — not necessarily fitness competitions but rather the way I have dedicated myself to a lifestyle and made choices to live the life that makes me perfectly happy.

Life is short. This your only chance to live the life you love. The sooner you realize this, the sooner you can adjust your choices accordingly. And forget about whether it happens early or late in your life. Age is just a number; it does not dictate what you are capable of. If I had listened to people about my age, I would have never started my fitness journey and would have passed up an experience that completely changed my self-esteem, my physical and mental health, and my vision of life. I congratulate myself every day for persevering according to what I believed to be good for me.

Be convinced that you can accomplish anything, because you never know what you can do until you try. Trust in the fact that you will succeed. Remember the example I gave earlier in the chapter: in the gym, I may think I will not be able to do something, but it is up to me to project only images of success in my head. Then I can do it. I will never lift the bar if I do not touch it. It is the same thing for all situations in life. Remember that you need not explain or justify what you feel is great for you. Your instinct knows what suits you the best, and you are the only one who will live your life. Find the courage to listen to yourself and to ignore the doubts of others. By taking the risk to discover your potential, you will only be surprised by how great you are!

04

GYM THERAPY

"Most days, it's not about building muscle, losing weight, or changing my body in any way. It's simply therapy for the heart, soul, and mind so I can tackle life head on with grace and grit."

BY: CASSIE LAMBERT

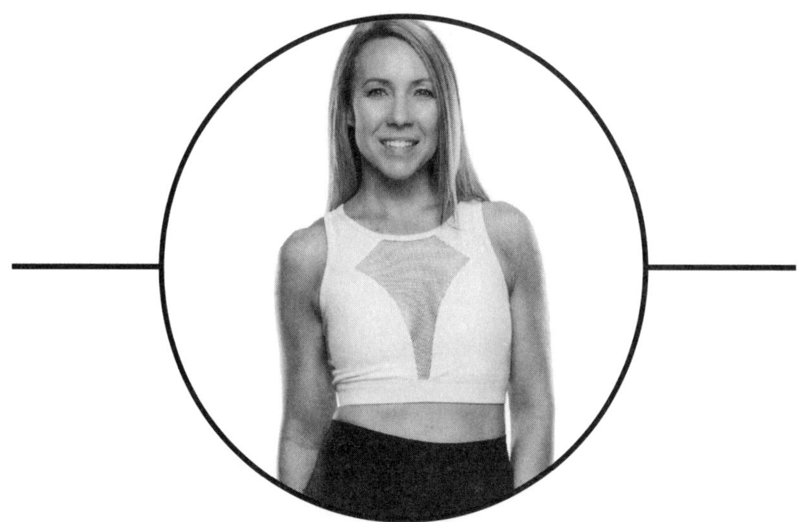

Cassie Lambert is an Army Veteran and a certified personal trainer specializing in helping women crush the weights with confidence. She has been published in *SELF, Oxygen, Men's Health*, and *SHAPE*.

While Cassie was born and raised in Michigan, as a military spouse, she is now calls a new place home every few years. She enjoys moving and exploring new places with her husband and three kids.

I once heard someone say that everyone needs a therapist, and part of me agrees. Talking with someone who can help you work through life's struggles is of great value. Personally, I believe that therapy can take a variety of shapes, though. I have found peace through a different form of one-on-one time: just me, a barbell in my hands, music in my ears, and some grit in my soul. It is here, alone and lost in my thoughts, that I have made it through the rocky road called life. I don't wear this as a badge of honor or mean to say that I have overcome every challenge in life on my own. What I know, however, is that without my gym therapy, I would not have made it through without a few more scars.

Of course, I did not always have this outlet. For years, I collapsed under the stress I placed on myself. I lashed out in anger at those closest to me, punched a few walls, and threw my phone down the street more times than I can remember. If I am honest, despite my carefree exterior, I felt lost and broken inside on most days. As a child, I never learned how to release my emotions, although this is due to no fault of my parents. I grew up in what many would consider a picture-perfect home. I had two loving parents who supported me in everything I did. There was not much, if any, fighting or yelling that I can recall. We spent most summers traveling to northern Michigan, spending time on the lake, laughing around a campfire, and roasting marshmallows. I cannot point to one specific event that made me so numb to my feelings. For many years, I just assumed that's who I was as a person. I viewed it as an irreversible characteristic — one I was not proud of but was also not necessarily interested in changing. One day when I was in college, I was conversing with my dad. I do not recall the exact reason for my anger on this particular day, but I remember him telling me not to resort to throwing my computer out the window. He said it in a joking manner, but I clearly had a track record for breaking things when life got a little too tough. I simply didn't know what to do when it felt like my world was spinning out of my control. The stresses of life, even minor ones, always weighed heavily on me. For many years, I felt as though there were a ticking time bomb living inside me, ready to explode. I hated this part of myself. I despised the fact that I would lash out and that I could not explain my anger.

But then all that changed.

I could have never predicted that a simple life decision would be the catalyst I desperately needed to change the anger I thought was intertwined in my soul.

BECOMING A SOLDIER

On September 11, 2001, I knew I needed to join the military. I was a senior in high school and was shocked by the images of the terrorist attacks on TV. Like so many other Americans on that day, I asked myself, "What can I do?" That day was my awakening to focus on something greater than myself, but the fear of not being strong enough to take on the physical demands of the military held me back.

Four years later, another graduation was upon me. This time, I was a senior in college at Michigan State University. Like everyone else, I was trying to figure out what I was supposed to do after graduation. I had spent more time drinking alcohol and going out with friends than studying during those four years, and nothing about the natural next phase of life, whether it is graduate school or a job in corporate America, excited me. I still felt that tug on my heart to finally join the U.S. Army. So one month after donning a cap and gown, I put on a different uniform and headed to basic training.

This life-altering decision would eventually push me into the weight room.

I quickly realized just how weak I was. Walking twelve miles with a thirty-five-pound rucksack on my back while wearing a suffocating weighted vest and carrying my rifle proved more difficult than I had imagined. While I made it through basic training, my personal performance quite embarrassed me. I shouldn't have been so shocked, given that my past as an "athlete" in high school saw me more likely to be riding the bench than picked for first string. I was active as a teenager but was never the fastest, strongest, or most agile on any of my sports teams.

I knew I had to make a change or risk being seen as a burden by my male counterparts once we deployed to Iraq. I was an interrogator, which meant I would likely be embedded with the infantry. Such an assignment would consist of long days and patrols in the hot sun with full gear, requiring strength and stamina I simply did not have.

I was completely lost the first day I stepped into the weight room, but it did not take long for me to fall head over heels for the weights. It was the thing I looked forward to doing at the end of each workday to de-stress and release all my thoughts and burdens. Every time I entered the weight room, I felt at peace, like I could exhale again after years of holding my breath. I felt alive and free from the time bomb that I once feared would go off inside me. I finally regained some control of my life, my emotions, and my sanity. It's as if places that were once dark inside me saw the light. With headphones on, I shut out the world around me and pushed through mental and physical barriers I didn't even know I had.

It was not long before I was in Iraq, newly married to my husband, who was deployed in Afghanistan at the same time. To be honest, nothing about the deployment scared me. I was ready, excited, and could not wait to go. After all, if I couldn't deploy, then what was the point of being in the Army? Why did I even join?

While I never feared for my life or safety, even in the most intense situations, I did experience moments of darkness during my year-long deployment. I was not prepared for death, nor was I prepared to see young soldiers who had little babies and families never return home with us. I was not as strong as I thought. Throughout that year, while most things were out of my control, one thing remained constant: the weights. I was no longer training for physical strength but rather for mental peace. My weight training gave me an ounce of normalcy among the uncertainty of day-to-day life in deployment. It was my place of therapy, comfort, and resiliency.

PREGNANCY

I was not sure how much I wanted to have kids until the moment I saw two blue lines on that pregnancy test. Motherhood was never something I felt called to do, but in a split second, everything changed. I became overwhelmed with emotion thinking of what my new life would be like in nine short months. It's strange how you can dream of and imagine your child before he or she is ever born. Somehow, those memories that have not yet occurred are already imprinted in your mind. Just as quickly as I felt joy, though, I felt pain like never before when I noticed blood on my pajamas eight weeks later. I knew in my gut what had happened before I even made it to the doctor the next day.

The pain of losing someone you loved so much but never had the chance to hold ran deeper than I could have imagined. It is impossible to describe how it feels to grieve all the things that never would come to be. I did not know how to move past the pain; I just knew I absolutely did not want to talk about it with anyone because talking just made things worse. I fell back on what I knew, on what I had learned to do when words were incapable of providing comfort. I turned back to the weights. My gym therapy grounded my thoughts and enabled me to work through the raw emotion of loss.

Just a little over two months later, I was blessed with a second chance to love. Of course, I asked my doctor even more questions this time around, especially about working out through pregnancy, and was given the green light to do what I was doing before. I ran right back to the place I knew would get me through the next nine months: the weights.

I hit the gym six days per week with a smile on my face, ready to train my body to carry this baby. "No days off" was my mindset until the baby was born. This mindset prepared me for what was ahead, and I felt strong and ready on the day of my delivery.

"This is what we trained for, kid," I whispered to my tummy.

Post-baby was no different. I went back to the thing that could help me get through this new part of my life. It was my new mama gym therapy, and I knew I would need it even more with my husband leaving shortly thereafter to South Korea.

MOTHERHOOD

It's funny. As mothers, we tell our children they can be anything, do anything, and achieve anything with hard work and drive. We tell them to reach for the stars, that they can have and do it *all.*

Then we turn around and say to ourselves:

I can't work out because I have kids.

I don't have time because of my kids.

I am too tired because of my kids.

What we are really saying to our children is that you can do anything, be anything, and achieve anything — until you have kids. Then you must put yourself on the back burner because their life, needs, and well-being should always come before your own.

Well, I'm saying that is a bunch of crap. I love my kids with every fiber in me, but to be at my best — to be able to love them, hold them, nurture them, provide for them, have patience with them, and laugh with them — I have to take care of me, unapologetically.

I will never forget the comments I received after my first son was born once others realized that gym time was a priority.

"You don't want to miss these moments."

"Just relax and enjoy these early years."

"You don't have to lose weight. Why do you work out so much?"

"There will be plenty of time for that later."

It was the last year of my Army service, and my husband had just left for South Korea six weeks after my son was born. Like any good mother would do, I dropped him off at daycare at 6am and picked him up around 5:30pm — and then yes, I went straight to the gym.

To many outsiders, this appeared selfish. Spending so many hours away from my newborn every day and choosing the gym over him didn't make sense to others. I see it quite differently. I was a new mom, by myself with absolutely no family around, trying to survive on no sleep with four or five feedings per night. Life was constant crying, rocking, and feeding, followed by more crying and more rocking. Maybe, if I was lucky, I could sleep for a few brief moments here and there.

The choices in front of me were simple: allow judgement from others to shame me into letting go of my gym therapy or unapologetically embrace who I was and what I needed in order to take care of myself so when the crying would not stop, when the sleep was non-existent, I could hold my son peacefully and stress-free. I chose the latter. I chose to love myself so I could love on him even more. I made sure I was mentally and physically fit enough to take care of him. Even if he did not know it, I was showing him that being a mom or dad does not have to be an excuse not to take care of yourself. My view did not change with baby number two, nor has it changed as they have grown up over the last several years. My boys know that Mama needs her gym therapy every week so she can be whole and present for them.

DOING LIFE

Not every day or every year is comprised of life-altering events, the kind that test your mental strength and resiliency. However, even on the simplest of days, life itself can be stressful. I want to be at my best to meet the demands of kids, work, and marriage. I don't want to snap at my family and friends because I have put myself and my needs last. I will not apologize for prioritizing "me time" by walking out the door before the sun comes up or when the sun sets, or sometimes even on vacations when others say to just relax. I know the old me; she is not far removed in my memory, and I don't want that anger or darkness to creep back in. So I take the time every week to work on me through my gym therapy.

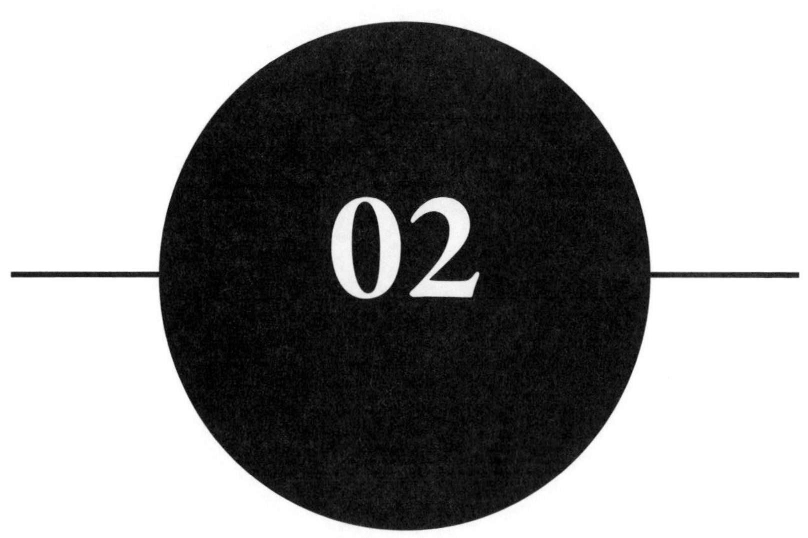

THE FREEDOM TO COMPETE IN A HEALTHY WAY

05

NOTHING TO LOSE

"Fitness is an inside job that manifests on the outside, not the other way around."

BY: JENA WEISS

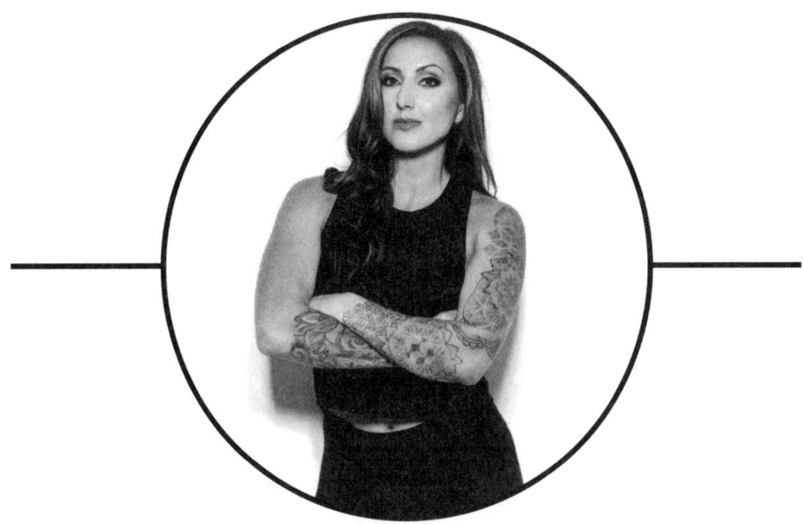

Jena Weiss is the owner of The Pound, a successful gym and training facility in upstate New York. With a clinical and social sciences in psychology degree from the University of Rochester, over ten years of experience as a certified personal trainer and strength coach, and a Level II Spirit Junkie Masterclass certification, she now works as a spiritual body and soul coach with a passion for helping others transform their lives from the inside out.

Jena is currently completing a teaching memoir titled *Fit to Love: My Journey from Self-Perfection to Self-Worth, with Nothing to Lose and Everything to Gain.* The book tells the story of a strength coach's journey through letting go of perfection, healing her childhood, and finding real love she didn't know she deserved. She has been featured in print in *Oxygen Magazine* and in online publications of *Muscular Development* and *RX Muscle.*

After decades of playing competitive sports, Jena quickly found a natural outlet in physical fitness after graduating from a prestigious college and finding herself unemployed. She navigated her way through success in fitness competitions, the body dysmorphic disorder and depression that followed, coaching, football, loss, and everything in between to establish herself as the coach she was destined to be.

Jena lives with her husband and their five labs(ish) on a two-hundred-acre farm in upstate New York.

Have you ever said to yourself, "If I could just lose ten pounds, then I'd be happy," only to find yourself a month down the road, ten pounds lighter with ten more to lose? Or maybe you've looked in the mirror to see yourself wearing that favorite pair of jeans you *swore* you'd get back into and yet you're still not happy.

As a gym owner and trainer for over ten years, I've worked with countless women seeking resolution through physical transformation. I've watched as they've met or even surpassed their goals, only to leave feeling the same or sometimes worse than they did before. I, too, have been guilty of this. Too often, we do not see where the real problem lies or that true healing is possible. I hope that in sharing my story, you will come to understand that if we are brave enough to dig up the problem beneath the surface, *freedom* is possible.

I can't do this.

I feel gross.

I'm going to look so fat.

These thoughts, accompanied by sheer angst, played on repeat in my mind as I tightly squeezed the "roll" protruding over the waistband of my favorite size-two jeans. It was a routinely hot Florida day in May of 2009, and I was riding in the back seat on the way to my very first photoshoot. I had just won the overall figure title at one of the largest bodybuilding competitions in the area a few weeks prior. In my mind, those few weeks made all the difference. In that short time, I had somehow gone from feeling stage-worthy to not being able to look at my reflection in the mirror. The disparity existed only in my mind; if I showed you the pictures from that photoshoot, you would see a girl with veins in her stomach, a girl who *must* be comfortable in her own skin. What I saw was nothing of the sort.

I weighed in at roughly one hundred and twenty-five pounds, but my days were consumed with compulsive thoughts about my body, ranging from how I could *feel* the fat on my stomach and legs jiggle when I ran to what I believed others were thinking or saying about me. I refused to wear shorts, even on the hottest Florida days, for fear of exposing the imaginary cellulite covering the backs of my legs. I avoided traveling home to see my family and often made excuses not to leave the house because the risk of going out and facing others was just too great.

There I was, with the perfect body that I just *knew* was going to solve all my problems — and with newly acquired depression and body dysmorphia and an eating disorder on the way.

That's the thing about trying to solve an internal problem with an external solution. It just will not work.

The large majority of women fight a very similar battle. No matter the story that led us here, somewhere along the way, we learned we were "not enough." We learned that in order to be loved, we must *do* something or *be* something that would make us worthy. If you're like me, or like the nearly half of Americans who report trying to lose weight in a given year,[1] at some point in your life, you probably thought losing weight or looking good was that something.

As the youngest of four girls left by our father to compete for our single mother's scarce attention, my story was that in order to be loved, I had to stand out. I learned a few core ways to do this: straight A's, athletic achievements, popularity, and physical appearance. After finishing school and eventually exhausting any lingering athletic options — even going so far as to subject myself to the Lingerie Football League — my physical appearance became the most favorable option.

In the beginning, I convinced myself that I had uncovered my true purpose in life through weight lifting and bodybuilding competitions. I fell in love with the freedom that initially came with my newfound confidence, and I was eager to help others discover that same feeling. Perhaps fitness did give me a feeling of freedom I had not previously experienced, but I still had a lot to learn.

When the stage lights went out and the attention faded, I found myself in one of the darkest places I have ever been in my life. I couldn't stand the sight of myself in the mirror, despite having a physical body that others admired, and my thoughts were a steady stream of relentless self-ridicule.

I spent about seven years on a roller coaster of extreme dieting and fitness competition highs, accompanied by the lowest of lows complete with hormonal imbalances and metabolic damage, disordered eating behavior, and depression. If I was preparing for a fitness competition, you would see a focused, driven, positive young woman

[1] Ducharme, J. (2018, July 12). About Half of Americans Say They're Trying to Lose Weight. Time Magazine. Retrieved from http://time.com/5334532/weight-loss-americans/

with a daily routine many looked upon with envy. My social media timeline was inundated with "progress pics" and filtered images of tuna and asparagus. Each post was an attempt to impress my "friends" and prove my worthiness of love, just as I had learned to do as a young girl. In the off-season, however, I was someone altogether different. I was overcome with shame and sadness. There were days I couldn't leave the house for fear of seeing someone I knew. You wouldn't hear from me on social media except for the occasional "throwback Thursday" photo, which became an excuse to post a past competition photo that was sure to get an influx of likes and comments: just enough validation to keep me afloat until the following Thursday.

It didn't matter if I was in prep mode or off-season mode, if I weighed one hundred and twenty-five pounds or one hundred and sixty-eight pounds (my heaviest): I felt the same inside. When I finally took an honest look at myself, I felt unworthy and unloved. The perfect body had fixed nothing because it wasn't my body that was broken.

Ironically, during this time in my life, I was also fully committed to helping others (primarily women) with their own physical transformations as a certified personal trainer and eventually a gym owner. Nearly every one of my clients hoped to alter something about her physical appearance, with the ultimate goal of feeling better about herself. What I had finally come to understand, however, was that no physical transformation would provide the healing they were seeking. It was not only possible for them to feel better *before* losing those ten pounds, it was *necessary*.

I was no longer willing to perpetuate the perfectionism and lies that had become the "fitness" industry. I didn't want to be another filtered face on social media, influencing women who were feeling less-than. I refused to promote another twenty-one-day fix or seven-day cleanse that I knew would leave my clients right back where they started. Knowing there was more to the equation, I was determined to do better. I simply couldn't continue to guide others if I was unwilling to let them see all of me: the things I had learned to love about myself but also my flaws, self-doubt, and insecurities; my successes but also my failures along the way.

I'm no Oprah, but one thing I know for sure is that feeling good in your body is an inside job that manifests on the outside, not the other way around. Six-pack abs will not make you feel good about yourself unless you *truly* feel good about yourself. That may seem like bad news at first glance, but trust me on this one, it's great news! It means you don't have to starve yourself or spend precious hours on a treadmill. It means the transformation you're after is far less about tracking every calorie and stride and far more about loving yourself and honoring yourself with choices and thoughts that serve you. You're probably thinking, "Sure, that sounds great, but how the heck do I do that?" I thought the exact same thing. Don't worry, I will not leave you hanging! If there's one thing that frustrates me, it's reading or hearing something insightful that fires me up but fails to provide any direction on how to get started, thus leaving me sitting on the couch with a slightly elevated heart rate.

I'm going to give you some exercises. I'm not talking squats or lunges but rather exercises for your mind and your soul to help you create subtle shifts that ultimately create lasting change in how you see and love yourself. What your trainer isn't telling you is that the transformation you seek, true *freedom*, is not available through fitness of the body alone but through fitness of the mind and soul as well.

However, while this work is simple, it isn't easy. I will give you some tools that have helped me, but it'll be up to you to put them to use, and that doesn't just mean pulling them out of the box every once in a while when something breaks. You'll need to use them daily, especially in the beginning, with the same frequency as those pesky negative thoughts you have. I'm guessing you've gotten so good at reminding yourself of all the reasons you shouldn't wear your favorite outfit or punishing yourself for taking one too many bites of the dessert you promised yourself you wouldn't have that you don't even notice when you're doing it anymore. The truth is, restrictive diets and excessive cardio routines are much easier than what I'm going to give you. These exercises will be tough, especially at first. As with any good workout program, you do the best you can. As you get better, you do better; consistency is key.

EXERCISE ONE: JOURNALING/FREE WRITING

There is so much power in putting pen to paper. Journaling and/or free writing is a great way to get your thoughts out, free from judgement, so you can take an honest look at all the thoughts creating your reality.

Fill in the blanks to complete these sentences in your journal:

I want to ____________________ so that I will feel ________ ____________________.

I don't feel _____________ now because _____________.

If I'm honest, I ______________________________.

Then set a timer for five or ten minutes and allow yourself to free write. This means putting the pen to paper and letting the words flow: no judgement, no filtering, no editing, just writing.

EXERCISE 2: MEDITATION

If the word meditation just threw you off in some way or you're thinking it's too woowoo, bear with me for a minute. I'm not saying you have to wear a robe or isolate yourself on a hilltop for days on end. Meditation can be as simple as sitting still for one minute. For some people, meditation happens during exercise. Keep an open mind and see what works for you.

WHAT DO I NEED TO HEAL MEDITATION

Arrange yourself comfortably in your personal space. You can sit up straight or lie down with your palms facing upward. Set a timer for five or ten minutes.

Begin by taking three deep breaths in through your nose and out through your mouth.

Repeat the following mantra throughout the meditation, allowing any thoughts or feelings to flow: *"What do I need to heal?"*

Return to the mantra any time you notice your mind starting to wander.

Close the meditation with three deep breaths, breathing in through your nose and out through your mouth.

Make notes in your journal of anything that came up for you. Stay alert throughout the day and over the next few days for any additional thoughts or experiences that may occur.

EXERCISE 3: AFFIRMATIONS

If you're anything like me, you have negative self-talk playing on repeat like a brand-new hit song. Unlike those hit songs, though, instead of reaching the point where you can't bear to hear it one more time, the negative talk just becomes background noise that you don't even notice. If we want to have any chance of shifting our mindset, we need to replace these negative thoughts with new, positive ones as often as possible. That means we have to do everything possible to keep our thoughts at the forefront of our minds. Here are three practices to increase your positive input.

1. Write one positive affirmation or mantra about yourself on a Post-it note and stick it to your bathroom mirror. Do this every day for a month.

2. Take your affirmation and design a colorful meme or picture that you can set as your phone background or lock screen. This will remind you of your new thoughts each time you glance at your phone. Change it out often so it doesn't just become a background you ignore!

3. Set an alarm or reminder in your phone to go off several times throughout the day. When the alarm goes off, create a habit of saying your affirmation out loud or to yourself. If you can, sit in stillness for one minute.

EXERCISE 4: GRATITUDE

We all spend far too much time focusing on all the things we have done wrong or all the ways we fell short. What would happen if we spent the same amount of time focusing on what we did right? I largely credit my gratitude practice for my transformation. I can trace back some of my most profound shifts to times when I was consistently practicing gratitude.

Begin or close each day by making a list of at least ten things you are grateful for and/or love about yourself.

EXERCISE 5: SOCIAL MEDIA DETOX

Set aside ten minutes to cleanse your social media pages. As you scroll through, take notice of what feelings come up. If any of the people you follow make you feel less-than or badly about yourself, whether you know them or not, click on those three little dots next to their name and then tap the bright red "Unfollow" button. Doesn't that feel good? Don't worry, that Instafamous fitness chick isn't going anywhere, and when you find yourself in a healthier place down the road, you can absolutely follow her again.

06

MAKING A COMEBACK

"Don't hide in the shadows of someone else's judgement or let someone else's insecurities define your life sentence. Instead look in the mirror and fall in love with the woman looking back at you, the woman who has survived so much and is stronger despite it all."

BY: ERICA GLASSFORD

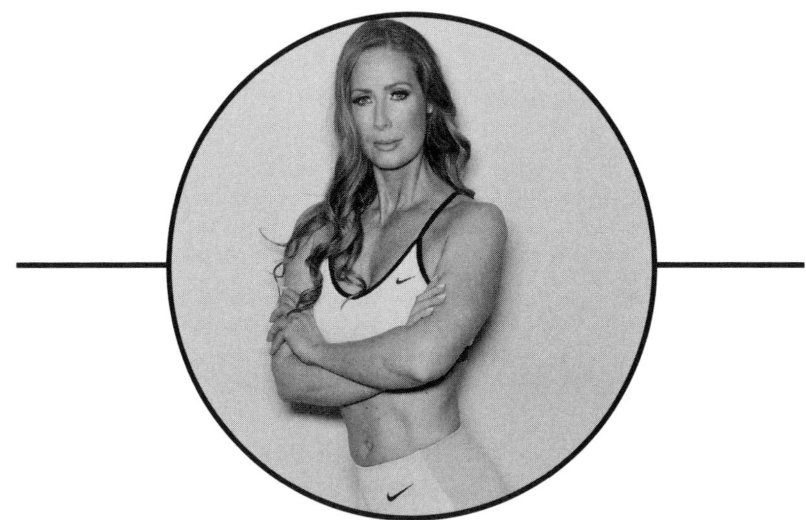

Erica is a certified nutrition coach, certified mindfulness coach, and certified lifestyle coach. She also holds titles as a Pro Masters Fitness Model and Grand Masters Bikini Champion. Originally from Seattle, Washington, she moved as a child to Canada with her parents and sister and now lives in a small hamlet just outside Calgary, Alberta with her family of five. Her most coveted title is that of Mom, and she takes every opportunity she can to cheer her kids on in their respective sports. In her spare time, she enjoys reading non-fiction history novels, hanging out with her two dogs, and indulging in the occasional night out dancing with her girlfriends.

www.ericabikinifit.com

fb: Erica Bikini Fit Nutrition & Lifestyle Coaching | ig: @erica_bikinifit

I had emotional breakdowns writing this chapter. Putting parts of my story out there was tough, and I tried to quit when it got too real. I would write a few words, delete them all, slam my computer shut, and walk away for a few days, only to come back and repeat the cycle. Why? Simple confidence issues. Absorbed in negative self-talk, I wasn't sure any part of my story deserved to be heard. *What if I suck? What could I possibly have to say that would inspire anyone? I am not "book-worthy."* These types of thoughts were exactly what I have been fighting so hard to teach other women to eliminate. I felt like a fraud, a walking contradiction: preaching self-love and forgetting to practice it.

Like most women, I have spent a good portion of my life not being comfortable in my own skin. My self-esteem ebbs and flows depending on the day; sometimes I see myself as a super-hot superhero mom of three, while other days I see myself as a bearded troll under the local bridge demanding junk food as payment to cross. I am not special, so why write my story? Then I was reminded by a fellow author that going through the ringer of life tends to provide some perspective. Although I waffle on my self-love from day to day, if I can learn to look in the mirror and more often than not fall in love with the woman looking back at me, maybe something in my journey will help you do the same.

My hot-and-cold self-esteem issues aside, I am the girl who cannot stand being told she can't do something. I am a goal-oriented person, defiant and competitive. In the past, however, my motives were often skewed by what I thought would make the people around me happy. I made choices that were not always healthy, mentally or physically. While I have always put a lot of pressure on myself, I used to give up when things didn't go my way. I sought approval from others, letting them define my self-worth. I let people treat me poorly and disrespect me, I didn't say no when I heard the knowing voice inside because I wanted to feel accepted, and I certainly didn't have the confidence to stand up for myself.

My story is not one full of adversity. It is a fairly common story filled with low self-esteem resulting in poor choices. It's a story of listening to the pressures of societal norms, looking for instant gratification to fill voids. The only adversity I needed to overcome was my own self-destructive behavior.

As far back as I can remember, I just wanted to succeed at something, to be something other than awkward and skinny. I was the stereotypical painfully shy, tall, skinny kid who got teased often. I constantly heard words like "anorexic" and "unhealthy," even though neither was true. While I already ate more than most, I was often pressured to eat more; it didn't matter what or how much I ate, though, I couldn't gain weight. Yeah, go ahead and curse me; I get it. I curse the younger me, too, because now I look at chocolate and it adds a dimple in my butt!

I was fifteen when my mom enrolled me in a self-improvement class at our local department store and I finally stood out in a good way. On the runway at our graduation fashion show, my height, which had once been a curse, became a blessing and my poise from years as a dancer showed well. My once awkward looks were now considered unique, and the instructor suggested that my mom take me to an open house at a local modeling agency. Like any insecure teenage girl looking for affirmation, I begged my mom until she agreed. Little did I know that pursuing this path would only fuel my insecurities.

Over the next few years, I went after modelling wholeheartedly; my parents cautiously encouraged me, thinking I was finally coming into myself. I was showing some outward confidence, and modeling seemed to fill that void of self-esteem I had lacked for so long. But it was a façade that did more damage than good in the long run, finally escalating to the point where I was acting like a high-rolling party girl on a half-assed contract in New York.

Then those crushing words: "You have potential, but your hips are a little big. You will need to lose five pounds before we will sign you."

Let me put this in perspective for you. I am five-foot-nine and I weighed a whopping one hundred and twelve pounds at the time. I had gone from being skinny-shamed to being told I was too fat. At this point, my appearance began to completely own me. I left that audition deflated and started on a diet of coffee and miracle weight loss cookies. The real miracle was that I fell for that marketing; they tasted like freakin' cardboard, and you didn't want to eat too many for fear of your colon combusting under the pressure! I didn't last much longer in the modeling world after that. It had worn me out with the partying and dieting, and I hit a wall. I called my folks crying and was on the next flight home.

My return from New York should have been the time to face reality and get a grip on my future. Instead I was on a one-way path to self-destruction, moving from bad choice to worse choice and eventually landing myself pregnant and in an abusive relationship. When he finally left me, I felt used, desperate, sure that my life was over. He had convinced me I would do no better than him and then kicked me to the curb for good measure. At that point, I said goodbye to any ounce of self-esteem I had left. Broken physically and emotionally, I was left standing on my parents' doorstep with a toddler.

We all have defining moments, and whether they are good or bad, they provide a lesson if you choose to see it. I have an amazing son because of that relationship; it also gave me the tools to educate all three of my children about the warning signs of an abusive relationship. I didn't always see things that way, though. I had to work hard to never fall victim to being a victim. I couldn't have done it without the support from my family and their understanding of the phases I went through. They had no problem adding a dose of love or reality when I needed it. After I had a small bout of misdirected emotional diarrhea, I remember my dad looking over his glasses and chuckling.

Me: "Dad, I am a twenty-five-year-old single mom with stretch marks. I live with my parents and I drive a four-door car. Who in their right mind would want this sort of baggage?!"

Dad: "Maybe you should take a harder look outside of that mirror and see what you have to offer."

I have never forgotten this conversation because it dawned on me that he was reminding me I was worth more than my exterior.

My confidence didn't come to me like a tsunami. It was more like pulling myself out of quicksand. I would gain some ground, but then I still had moments when I walked around looking at my feet. Years of feeling like I was not good enough were tough to erase, and it wasn't until much later that I figured out my inner sass was buried just under the surface, waiting to escape once I felt safe.

It was a long journey to find that girl, a journey complicated by normal life events such as my second and third pregnancies. I realized that every moment of those pregnancies was a miracle and I wanted so badly to be that glowing pregnant woman, but that was not my destiny. The changes in my body were a challenge. I struggled with how I looked yet continued to eat everything I could find. Pregnancy equaled depression, which only compounded my emotional eating.

Please don't hate me after you read this next sentence. Even with the pregnancy weight I gained from all that food, I was lucky enough to go back to being lean after I gave birth. Notice I said "lean" and not my "pre-baby body." There is no going back to that without some aftermarket modifications! Every morning I roll up what is left of the mounds of skin that once were beautiful boobs but now resemble dirty sweat socks with nipples, and let's not even discuss the dog jowls that appear in my midsection every time I bend over! Bottom line: for years, I took my metabolism for granted and comfortably ate whatever I wanted. I ate out of boredom, to comfort myself, and even to fill a void, realizing but not worrying that I was slowly gaining weight; after all, it had taken no effort to lose weight in the past. I didn't realize how much I had let myself go until I saw a picture of my backside that made my retinas burn. Horrified at the sheer landscape of my butt and the Michelin man rolls hanging out of the back of my bra, I wondered just how and when this had happened. This horrifying moment is where my fitness journey began.

I didn't jump right into the gym. It intimidated me. Instead, I started with walking; then once I had some new-found motivation, I went back to my old running days. Running with my mom-bod posed an entirely new set of problems . . . like the fact that running and breathing at the same time made tears run down my legs. Despite the fear that someone might notice my wet running tights or find out the reason for my excessive bathroom breaks, I joined a local running group. I found my competitive spirit during sprint training (I was not going to let a boy beat me!), and during hill training I sang and told everyone that each hill was a "mound of opportunity." After years of throwing myself into work and family, I was really finding *me* again. Somehow by taking care of my outside, my inside was slowly gaining strength, too. I began to set goals for myself. Before I knew it, I was running half marathons regularly and even managed to run a full marathon.

My fitness journey may have begun with a desire to look better naked, but it morphed many times over the years. The first big change in my attitude toward fitness came when I watched my daughter struggle with crippling anxiety. Suddenly I realized that she could be me as a child and that she needed me to fight for her until she could learn to fight for herself. My kids are my world, and watching any of them struggle with confidence like I did was terrifying. Losing my favorite aunt to cancer added to my change in attitude. I had already watched my grandma pass from complications with diabetes, and when I lost my aunt, I started reflecting on some family patterns. A number of relatives on my mom's side struggled with late onset diabetes. Would I face the same destiny as I aged? What legacy was I going to leave for my children? I didn't want that life for myself or my kids. My fitness journey was no longer about how I looked; it became about being strong mentally and defying family history.

Unlimited cardio was my jam and I had lost quite a bit of weight with it, but I still had high body fat and not much muscle definition. The gym still intimidated me, and I was fearful of looking bulky if I lifted weights. It wasn't until a close friend who was training for her first bikini competition invited me to train alongside her for moral support that I put my fears aside. Lifting weights was like an epiphany for me. I saw muscles that I didn't know existed. It inspired me to train a little harder, and at the age of forty-one, I decided to get in the best shape of my life.

My journey transformed once again when I decided to tackle my first fitness competition just to prove a point. I overhead a rant about how "bikini competitors are not athletes, that they are doing it out of vanity and did not portray true strength." It was uneducated and judgmental, and although I had not originally set out to compete when I started lifting weights, that little speech was all the motivation I needed. Four months later, I stepped on that stage for the first time *as an athlete.*

Stepping on stage had some side effects for me. It gave me a sense of accomplishment outside of my "normal" life and showed me how fighting through all the tough parts of prep built more confidence and self-awareness. It got me over my fear of being judged by complete strangers. However, one of the most interesting side effects of competing is that my opinion of vanity has changed. My original attitude was that vanity was a bad thing, but now that I am well into what I like to call my "fuck-it forties," I make no apologies for coming across a bit boastful now and then. I have worked hard to get where I am, and I think more women need to be proud and stop defaulting into apology when they show confidence. I try to live by the famous Abraham Hicks quote: "People will love you, people will hate you, and none of it will have anything to do with you."[2] Not that I don't still waffle from time to time and fall into the trap of letting others' judgement momentarily affect me, but mostly I have learned to let those things go. Loving myself will *always* be a process.

Despite all my success with competing and the opportunities it has brought me, I still don't see myself as anything other than an average mom of three. Only now, I am a mom with muscles and a stronger mind. In my spare time, I use my warped sense of humor to address some real issues and stigmas we women face via social media; somehow that has gained me a loyal following, defining me as an influencer. This doesn't change the fact that I still yell at my kids and scrub toilets. Being an influencer is uncharted territory for me, but I hope that by putting myself out there and sharing more of myself publicly, I can inspire other women to step outside their comfort zone, stop apologizing, and learn to love themselves through every stage of their journey. Breaking through your own threshold of fear and judgement is beautiful and empowering.

[2] Goodreads. (2019). Abraham Hicks quotes. Retrieved from https://www.goodreads.com/quotes/791609-people-will-love-you-people-will-hate-you-and-none

If I can give you anything to take with you, it's this: start taking care of yourself sooner. Don't wait for your fuck-it forties; start with your tough-shit twenties or sooner. Someone will always have an opinion about how you eat, work out, talk, dress, look, and sometimes breathe, but whether you give a shit or not is ultimately up to you. All too often, we get caught up in taking care of our families or get lost in our careers and forget to live our best life. We lose our identity in being a mom or a wife, and we dwell on the bad situations we faced in our past. You may have had setbacks in your life, but bad situations are everywhere. Do not let them define you. Instead, define yourself by your comebacks.

07

THE POWER OF PERSISTENCE

"Fall in love with the journey,
and the result will just be a bow on top."

BY: ANNIE GRAFT

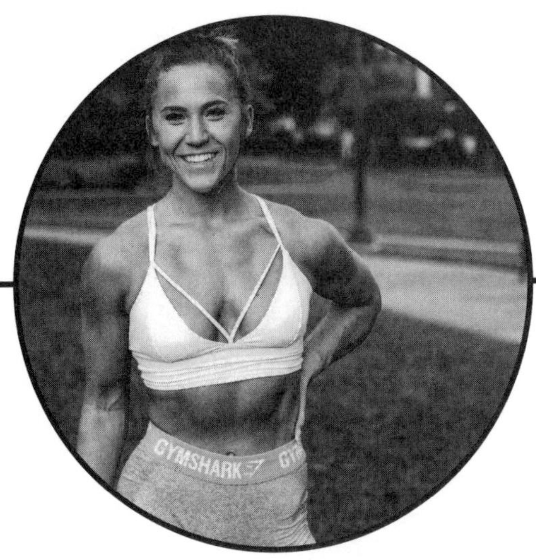

Annie Graft is twenty-three years old and currently lives in Texas. She grew up in the suburbs of Chicago as the middle child of three. She attended college at the United States Air Force Academy in Colorado Springs, Colorado and commissioned into the USAF. As an active duty Air Force officer, Annie works full-time as a Public Affairs officer while running her own online coaching business, personal brand (Fit Life Fit Me), workout app, and health and wellness company. She is passionate about inspiring people, predominantly women, to ditch their excuses and embrace their best lives.

Fitness is easy when you're young. Your parents make your lunches, sign you up for activities, and set you up with play dates. Things aren't up to you, and even if they were, you have all the time and energy in the world. Being active isn't something you have to think about consciously. Running is a natural instinct when you're nine years old. Ice cream is okay because you haven't yet learned that it makes you bloated. You don't associate the *feeling* of being full with that voice telling you that you *are* fat.

Fitness isn't a requirement when you're a child; it just *happens* somehow. It isn't something you spend the majority of your day stressing about. The number on the scale is something only the doctor pays attention to. The reflection in the mirror is only studied when you're trying to pull your hair up into a ponytail without your mom's help. The bathing suit in your drawer is a symbol of summer fun, not something that causes you stress.

Until it is.

For me, that happened in the fifth grade when my gymnastics coach called me fat.

I had always been an active kid. My after-school activities consisted of soccer practice, dance lessons, frog-catching, tree-climbing, and gymnastics. Before long, gymnastics required such a vast amount of time that the other sports and activities fell to the wayside. Gymnastics became my passion. I was a competitive soul, but I didn't just compete with the other girls for better meet scores, placements, and rankings. From as early as I can remember, inside the privacy of my own head, I was also competing for a body that wasn't deserving of the title "fat." I constantly compared myself to the girls around me.

Her legs don't touch when she stands with her feet together . . .

Her thighs don't wiggle when she runs down the vault runway . . .

Her stomach doesn't pouch out when she waits for her turn on the balance beam . . .

Before I reached the age of thirteen, I believed that, for some reason, my body wasn't "good enough." Whether these lies were coming from the mouth of my coach or from that tiny voice inside my head, I had come to believe them at an early age. This went on for years. I went on a diet in sixth grade because I truly thought I was fat.

I believed that if I lost weight, I would be prettier, happier, and better at gymnastics. It consumed my every thought.

Years later, this belief was still affecting me in serious ways. I remember sitting in my dorm room after a week of only consuming cucumber juice and lemon/cayenne pepper shots, finishing off a jar of peanut butter by the spoonful and thinking that *maybe one day* I could stop. *Maybe one day I could stop obsessing over the way I look and just be HAPPY.*

It seemed impossible.

After nearly a decade of struggling with disordered eating and body image issues, I retired from the gymnastics world, which left me to deal with my struggles alone. During my junior year of college, I had to find fitness for myself: without gymnastics, without a coach yelling at me, without someone forcing me to do it. I had to find what fitness meant for me, Annie Graft, outside of the sport that had once consumed my life.

This is where my story really starts.

At first, the amount of equipment in my college gym overwhelmed me. So much metal. It scared me. I recruited my roommate to come with me so I didn't have to be the only girl in the weight section. The inner voice that had controlled me for twenty-one years insisted that I would mess up, I would use a machine wrong, I would have terrible form, all of which would cause my fellow gym-goers to laugh, point, and talk behind my back. Despite my self-consciousness, though, I knew that if I let that fear stop me, it would be impossible to improve in the ways I wanted.

I had placed a mental limit on my ability to succeed in the gym because I worried about others' opinions. I didn't realize that everyone around me was just focused on themselves. It happens to the best of us! We think that "Becky" on the other side of the gym is whispering about our bad form, our out-of-shape body, our raggedy old shorts when really, she's asking her friend if you can tell she's wearing a pad under her leggings. We need to get out of our own heads and realize that if we want to become better versions of ourselves, we cannot allow the fear of judgement to hold us back. This is one of the first lessons that the gym taught me, and boy, has it been useful!

I found that when I followed a plan, the vastness of the gym was much less intimidating. Having a plan also kept me coming back, day after day. It made the gym a non-negotiable because I knew there was work to be done and I didn't have an excuse to skip it. I kept my head down, headphones in, and was on a mission. Your fitness plan might entail getting a gym buddy, someone to hold you accountable and keep you company in the gym. It might mean laying out your gym clothes the night before so you don't give yourself an excuse to skip your workout altogether. Whatever your plan is, I encourage you to find a way to make the gym a mandatory part of your day! The first daily workout plan I committed to was Kayla Itsines' twelve-week Bikini Body Guide. I loved having a plan, challenging myself, and seeing results from hard-ass work. I never skipped a day.

I fell love with fitness in a smelly, stuffy, college-kid-packed gym using nothing but dumbbells and my bodyweight. It doesn't have to be fancy, y'all. I know Instagram glamorizes fitness and makes us think we have to have all the newest workout gear, the most advanced supplements and macronutrient calculation, the most intense trainer and lifting plan . . . But I am here to tell you differently. I am here to reassure you that your XL t-shirt is more than okay. The fact that you moved your body and got yo' sweat on is what matters. Don't wait for perfection to start. Don't wait for a sign to start. Don't wait for the "right time" to start . . . *Just start.*

Falling in love with fitness opened the door to a life filled with challenges, successes, failures, and more growth than I could have ever imagined. I realized that by pushing myself in the gym, getting through physically difficult workouts, and showing up the next day to do it all again, I proved to myself that I, Annie Graft, am capable of enduring tough things outside of the gym, too. *Wow.* That is powerful, and it is true for everyone in this world.

You, my friend, are capable of pushing through hard times, too, however they show up in your life: facing an emotional breakup, a financial loss, or an injury or sickness, getting fired from your dream job, losing a friend, or even just making a difficult decision. It may seem silly but working on yourself and transforming your health and fitness will show you that you *can* push past it all. Setting a goal, working toward it every day despite the hard times that arise, and then conquering that goal is a priceless journey, one that will teach you lessons for a lifetime.

The thing is, though, it is *so easy* to simply set a goal. I bet if you're reading this right now, you have set a fair share of goals in your life. Let me tell you, it is an entirely different beast to actually make that goal happen. Most people reading this will set goals all day long but never do anything about them. Don't let that be you! Do not set a goal, write it down, and then trash it when things get hard on day five because you're tired and your legs are so sore that you cannot even sit on the toilet. (Trust me, sis, we've all been there.) Do not be someone who wants more out of life but is unwilling to put in the work to see any real results.

The biggest belief I have in this world is that everyone — yes, everyone — is capable of achieving greatness. Sis, just because Becky over there is achieving greatness does *not* mean there is any less greatness for you to achieve in your own capacity. We all bring different talents and passions to the table; that's the beauty of life! The only difference between you and Becky is that she hasn't quit on herself.

Despite eight knee surgeries, a gymnastics career cut short, a failed attempt at my first bikini prep, and many more failures that would take too long to tell, I did not give up. I will never give up because I learned early in my fitness journey that giving up on yourself does absolutely nothing. Quitting on leg day because it's hard and you're tired doesn't help you. It only hurts you. And giving up on yourself during those hard moments in life does the same.

Don't get me wrong. Just because I overcame challenges while learning these lessons does not mean that I do not still endure challenges. I definitely still have hard times when I find it nearly impossible to push on. But the lessons I learned from walking into the gym even though I had no idea what I was doing, sweating my butt off at 4am when nobody else showed up, getting back on the beam even when I had face-planted moments earlier . . . those are the same lessons that have encouraged me when I started my personal business two years ago, when I struggled with depression and addiction and didn't want anyone to know, and when I thought I was losing the love of my life (my now-fiancé.) These lessons have changed my life for the better, and it is all because I refused to quit on myself even in the darkest of moments.

Wherever you are in your journey right now, I challenge you to set some goals that scare the shit out of you. Set goals that might seem crazy impossible. Set goals that you're scared to say out loud. And from there, break it down day by day. After that, it's only a matter of never quitting.

You're in full control, sis. So what's your next move?

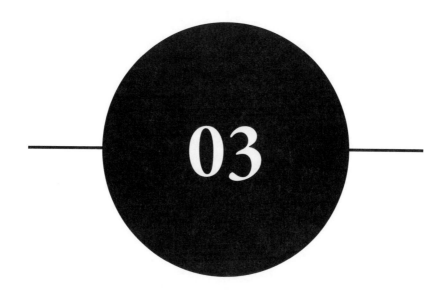

THE FREEDOM TO TRANSFORM

08

HOWE FOOD SAVED ME

"Nothing works unless you do."

BY: AMY HOWE

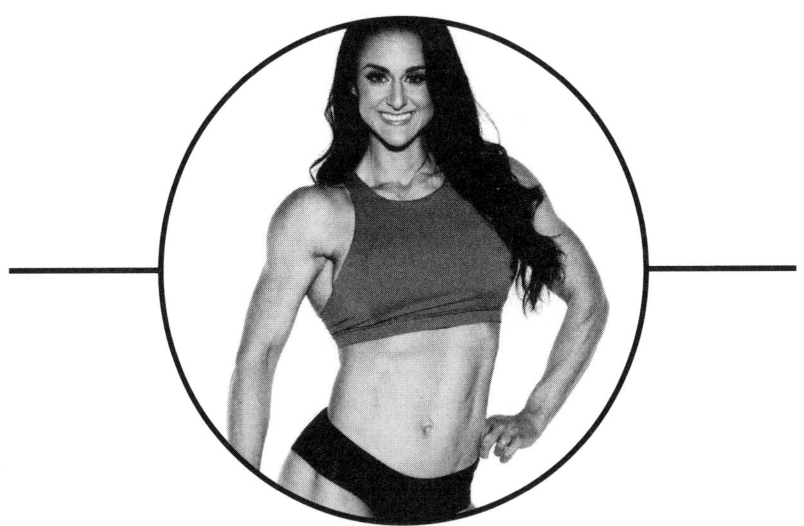

Amy Howe is the proud mother of beautiful four-year-old boy named Danden, as well as a passionate dog lover, caring wife, entrepreneur, personal trainer, coach, business mentor, fitness competitor, author, published fitness model, and body transformation coach. She has dedicated her life to bettering others by sharing her passion for balanced nutrition and flexible dieting strategies and her love for fitness.

At the young age of nineteen, Amy started her business, Howe Fit, out of the trunk of her car. She has worked countless hours to help her community thrive through volunteering as a public speaker, serving as a liaison for local school boards to educate young students about entrepreneurship, creating a safe environment for her Howe Fit members, mentoring her online clients, and serving as a friend with advice or help when anyone is in need. Becoming sober and free from alcohol and disordered eating created a clear path for Amy's journey to become the woman and leader she always knew she could be. With this new lifestyle and a growing passion for health promotion and balanced and flexible nutrition strategies, she became Howe Fit inside and out.

Website: amy.howe.fit

fb: @Amy Howe | ig: @amyhowefit

Head at the bottom of a food-filled toilet bowl, with puke-stained teeth, rotten breath, and raw fingers, I knew I had hit rock bottom. How could this be my life?

I was afraid of food. I feared every single thing I put in my mouth, whether healthy or indulgent.

I just wanted to be thin, pretty, successful, and accepted. I knew I needed to make a change, not only for myself but also because I had become a hypocrite. Every day, I was preaching to my clients to eat, work out in moderation, enjoy life, and be healthy. All the while, I was working ninety-plus hours and exercising over twenty hours a week, fueled on limited sleep and remnants of food and vodka.

How could I be a leader when I couldn't even look at food without wanting to vomit immediately? Who was I to preach about health when I was the most depressed and unhealthy person I knew?

With tears streaming down my face, hair matted in my signature pineapple up-do, eyes staring down at my wasted, chewed-up twelve-inch chicken sub, I knew things could not get worse than this.

It was like a spark went off in my head, that light bulb moment you hear people talk about in the movies but never think you will experience yourself. Without question, I had that magical moment on February 20, 2013. This chapter of my life I would label as "Not Who — But Howe Am I?" A re-birth, a transformation from something damaged to something beautiful and whole took place that day. I sat on this and thought long and hard about how I wanted my life to play out and who I really wanted to be. This conversation with myself reignited my passion for health and knowing my self-worth. *Finally,* for once I would not put others before myself as I had done for so long. I would make myself a priority. This clear vision of what I wanted for my life helped me pursue my dreams and achieve my goals:

1. to be healthy;
2. to have a good relationship with food;
3. to not feel the need to be perfect all the time based on society's impossible standards of what personal trainers or women *should* look like;

4. to be successful both financially and personally in my relationships with family, friends, and most importantly myself; and
5. to actually like what I see when I look in the mirror.

I knew that turning my life around would not consist of just one or two little steps in the right direction; it would take a complete overhaul of the person I currently was. This extended to my daily ritualistic behaviors, my food thoughts, my negative self-talk, my views on relationships, my hobbies and habits, and my toxic friendships.

How does one start over?

If we start the process of change by developing a clear plan to do something different than we have done the previous week, it won't matter how small our efforts. If we just start this miracle transformation process and commit to changing ourselves, then everything changes. And here's what is interesting: the difference between failure and success is subtle.

Let me explain by giving you *my* definitions of failure and success.

Failure. This concept is so much more complex than just being unsuccessful at something. I define failure as a few errors in judgment repeated every day due to a lack of care or overall vision.

Now here is my definition of *success*: a peace of mind, an attitude that you embody. Success doesn't mean being rich or famous; rather, it speaks to small yet important disciplines practiced every single day.

When you look at successful people, you will almost always discover that they have a plan behind their success. They know what they want, they work out a foundation for success within a considered strategy, and they take the necessary steps to reach their objectives.

In 2013, after my light bulb moment, I decided it was time to get even more serious with my goals and sign up for my first fitness show. Perhaps a bold move given my body abuse in the past, but I was up for an extreme challenge and with the help and support of my coach and now great friend, Mike Cardoso, I figured what did I have to lose?

I had always imagined myself up on stage, but the thought of giving up alcohol, my social existence, and essentially what I saw as my identity (my way of life) had been something I could not bring myself to commit to. But I believe all things happen in your life at the correct time, and I now welcomed this challenge as an opportunity to become my best self yet.

Over sixteen weeks of intense physical and mental training, Mike opened my eyes to the importance of proper fuel in the form of real food. He showed me that eating the right types of food in the correct amounts could help me achieve my goals far more quickly than restriction, deprivation, and purging.

Finally on a balanced eating plan, I was seeing results week after week: defined abs, sculpted shoulders, less cellulite on my hips and thighs. I also experienced so many other benefits from the proper nourishment. My hair and nails grew longer and stronger, my skin had become clearer and more lifelike, my energy soared, and I had mental clarity like never before, laser-like focus, and banished anxiety.

I credit my transformation to food, competition, my coach Mike, and most importantly, to me for allowing myself to be worthy of this positive change. However, when I tell people that competing helped *cure* my eating disordered past, they are almost always shocked. As a coach and friend of several fitness competitors, I've seen how seemingly healthy and happy competitors almost always end up with poor self-image issues and distorted eating troubles and have a hard time accepting their body when it transitions back to normal post-show. I will admit, after having completed seven shows now, it gets harder and harder to transition into a healthy off-season of higher body fat; you get used to feeling on top of the world when you are lean, confident, and what you consider your "best self." But I also know now that staying at those scary, unhealthy, and unrealistic low body fat percentages is unsustainable at best and is devastating long-term, both mentally and physically.

Do you need to compete to reach your goals as an average man or woman? Absolutely not. Losing weight, building muscle, and cutting fat doesn't start by grabbing a dumbbell at the gym, buying new workout gear, or getting fresh kicks. It starts in your head with a simple decision to try.

FOUR STEPS TO HELP YOU COMMIT TO YOUR GOAL

1. Get your mindset right. Success in any aspect of life starts with your mindset. A positive attitude can go a long way toward helping you to deal with life's daily drudgeries more effectively. Positive thinking brings a whirl of optimism into your life and helps you to stay inspired and energized along the way.

2. Refine your goals. It's hard to commit yourself to something if your finish line is not defined and within reach.

3. Focus on what's important. Time and energy are precious but limited resources. It's easy to get caught up in forever responding to the things that seem most urgent, rushing from one commitment to the next. To prevent this, identify what is most important to you within a short-term timeframe.

4. Hold yourself accountable. Being accountable means more than just being responsible for something. It's also ultimately being answerable for your actions. To hold yourself accountable, you must find the motivation to do difficult things and put yourself at the top of your priority list among all of life's daily to-dos.

Since deciding to hang up my competing heels in May 2018, I have embraced a little more flexibility within my life in terms of my personal nutrition strategies. I have learned through my personal struggles, as well as years of working with clients, that deprivation, elimination, and restrictive diets almost always end with a lack of adherence, resulting in failure. Instead, the style of eating I practice and preach on the daily is called "Flexible Living through Macronutrients."

A Flexible Living Macronutrient eating style goes a step further than typical calorie counting to count macronutrients — grams of proteins, carbs, and fats. Learning how to count macronutrients takes some effort, but it's a method that anyone can use and benefit from, regardless of age, gender, activity level, or fitness goals.

USE THE FOLLOWING STEPS TO GET YOU STARTED.

1. Figure out your calorie needs. To get started, you must determine your overall caloric needs. You can either use a simple online calculator, like the *Freedieting.com* online calorie counter, or the Mifflin-St. Jeor equation:

Men: calories/day = 10 x weight (kg) + 6.25 x height (cm) – 5 x age (y) + 5

Women: calories/day = 10 x weight (kg) + 6.25 x height (cm) – 5 x age (y) – 161

Then multiply your result by your activity factor, a number that represents different levels of activity:

Sedentary: x 1.2 (limited exercise)

Lightly active: x 1.375 (light exercise fewer than three days per week)

Moderately active: x 1.55 (moderate exercise most days of the week)

Very active: x 1.725 (hard exercise every day)

Extra active: x 1.9 (strenuous exercise two or more times per day)

Calories can either be added or subtracted from your total expenditure in order to reach different goals. In other words, those trying to lose weight should consume fewer calories than they expend, while those looking to gain muscle mass should increase calories.

2. Decide on your ideal macronutrient breakdown. After determining how many calories to consume each day, the next step is to decide what macronutrient ratio works best for you.

Typical macronutrient recommendations are:

Carbs: thirty to fifty percent of your total calories

Fats: twenty to thirty-five percent of total calories

Proteins: twenty-five to thirty-five percent of total calories

Keep in mind that these recommendations may not fit your specific needs; your ratio can be fine-tuned to achieve specific objectives.

3. Track your macros and calorie intake. The term "tracking macros" means logging the foods you eat on a website or app or in a food journal.

4. Implement balance within your food choices. Am I on point with my nutrition one hundred percent of the time? No, I am human and have weak moments here and there just like the rest of us. I want my clients to be happy and successful and to find a sustainable method of living. To help them accomplish this, I promote an 80/20 balance within your food choices. This is an approach to healthy eating that teaches you balance, moderation, and indulgence without guilt. The basic idea of the 80/20 rule is very simple. In order to be healthy and balanced, you don't have to make healthy food choices one hundred percent of the time. Developing the skill of flexible restraint, which is the ability to moderately control your eating, is important to weight-loss success. The key is to find the balance between control and flexibility so that your eating plan is not so rigid that it is impossible to stick to. The macronutrient method of eating provides a system for having treats and indulgences without sacrificing weight loss or long-term happiness.

Whatever method you decide on to help achieve your goals, keep in mind that your ultimate goal should always be your health. Good health is not something you can buy; it is something you must cultivate daily.

09

KEEP MOVING: FINDING THE BLESSING IN EVERY LESSON

"Optimal performance requires holistic health, which means caring for the mind, body, and soul."

BY: HEATHER LEE CHAPMAN

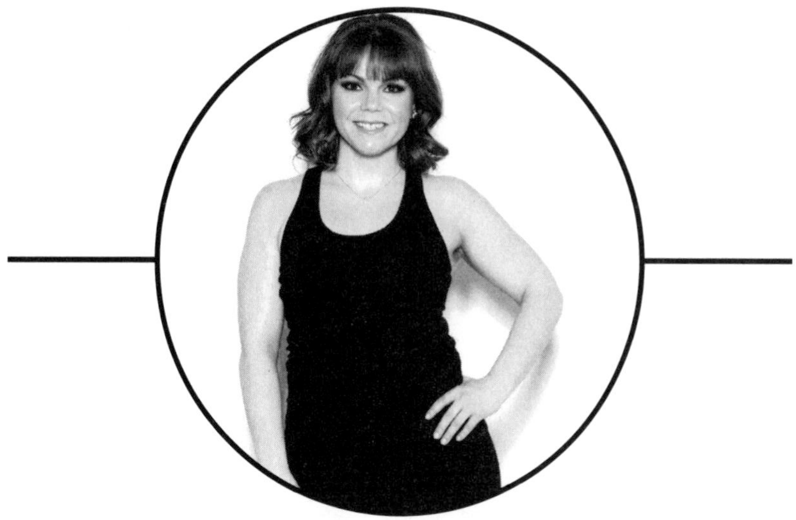

Heather Lee Chapman is a personal success coach with over a decade of experience coaching individuals to be their best and live their best lives through mindset, movement, and nutrition. She is a certified nutritional practitioner with a diploma in applied nutrition, as well as a personal trainer specialist. Heather has a bachelor's degree with honors in human kinetics, with a major in movement science and minors in biology and social sciences. She is a lifestyle and brand ambassador for Arbonne and an affiliate for the Proctor Gallagher Institute.

Heather is also the creative director of HLChealth.com and an inspiring educational speaker. She believes that we are all meant for greatness and for a fulfilled and happy life, and her mission is to ensure we all achieve those goals. Heather believes it is essential that you treat the body as a whole: mind, body, and soul. She has worked with many individuals from athletes to individuals with brain injuries and spinal cord injuries to improve their quality of life and can assist you in identifying areas of improvement for optimal physical and mental performance. She focuses on identifying limiting beliefs and replacing them with affirmations and actions that serve you, recreating yourself to align with your truth, step into your power, and identify your true passion and purpose.

For some people, fitness is life; for others, exercise is scary or next to impossible. Regardless of how you feel about fitness, it's important to find a way to move that works for you. Movement is freeing; it increases circulation and brings nutrients and oxygen through the blood to your whole body. Movement also increases your happy hormones. Your movement practice could be Tai chi, dancing, organized sports, joint mobility training, walking, running, yoga, chair yoga, stationary biking, outdoor biking, or swimming or water exercises. Whatever it is, just get moving and feel alive.

For me, movement makes me feel free as a bird. Sports and fitness have always been a huge part of my life. I started swimming at a young age and was obsessed with figure skating because of its balance between physical challenge and creativity. In high school, I could be found choreographing my own dances in the kitchen, and I loved playing soccer and basketball because of the team atmosphere and competitive challenge. Movement was my outlet; when I was upset and didn't know how to express myself, I would run. When I was overly excited and full of energy and didn't know what to do with it, I would work out. It became my cure for everything. Late in high school, I took a fitness class and discovered that I had a major passion for fitness. The dream of being a personal trainer and owning a business entered my mind.

My passion is to help people own their lives through mindset, movement, and nutrition and have spent the last decade expanding my knowledge of human performance and potential to help people heal holistically. I believe that a holistic approach to health is key! I have learned this from my own life experience as well. I had multiple health issues growing up: allergies, digestive disturbances, mood issues, and more. When I was twelve, I took part in a study at the University of Toronto that observed the relationship between food and behavioral issues, bladder issues, and digestive issues. Based on my results, doctors recommended that I go on a no-sugar and no-dairy diet. The transformation in my body, behavior, fitness levels, and overall health that year was astonishing. If I showed you before-and-after pictures, the before shots would look like an inflated hot air balloon. I became obsessed with fitness and nutrition and started counting calories and weighing myself until it reached an unhealthy point. I needed to find a balance between being healthy and accepting myself for who I was.

After an injury in high school, I couldn't exercise like I had before. In addition, I was not eating the way I should have been. I put on all the weight I had lost and more. A few months into studying at university, I decided it was time to make a change. This time I was determined to lose weight the right way, the healthy way, to be fit and stay fit. I set a plan: I would only eat what made me feel good (healthy, not for pleasure) and I would exercise six days a week. Soon this plan became an obsession again. I lost all the weight again yet still saw myself as overweight.

Shortly after university, I started to realize that I was not well. I would wake up swollen, in pain, with massive digestive upset, low mood, and irritability. I suffered multiple head traumas and back injuries that stopped me in many areas of my life. In search of answers, I found them through studying nutrition (The Institute of Holistic Nutrition), neuro-anatomy training (Z Health Education), and the power of the mind (The Proctor Gallagher Institute). I learned that I had leaky gut, a hormonal imbalance, adrenal fatigue (also known as burnout), and nutrient deficiencies. I also had visual and vestibular imbalances, muscular imbalances, jammed joints, and old injuries that were affecting my movement. I realized I had an unhealthy self image from struggling with health issues most of my life. My limiting beliefs and negative self-talk were affecting my ability to heal. I went on a mission to heal myself and share my new-found knowledge with my clients and fellow healthcare practitioners.

YOUR GUT

Leaky gut can affect your digestion, allergies, auto-immune responses, inflammation responses, nutrient absorption, energy levels, mood, cognitive function, and more. Due to my leaky gut and the related malabsorption issues, I was lacking many macro and micronutrients, which caused a lot of my symptoms. To heal my gut, I needed to remove the factors contributing to the symptoms. I went on an anti-inflammatory diet: no dairy, processed sugars, gluten, coffee, alcohol, or other inflammatory foods. I had to rebalance my gut flora by using anti-bacterial, anti-fungal, and anti-parasitic herbs, supplements, and food to kill the overgrowth of bad bacteria throughout my body. I used probiotics and probiotic foods to re-inoculate the good bacteria and liquid vitamins and mineral supplements to replace what my body was lacking and heal the lining of my digestive tract.

It's hard to want to exercise when you don't feel well because of malnutrition, digestive disturbances, inflammation, allergic reactions, skin irritations, and itchiness. You may feel more lethargic, slower, and weaker, affecting your overall performance. When you're constantly bloated, which can happen with leaky gut, it is hard to contract your core properly. This causes unwanted tension in areas of the body. Inflammation can also make it painful to move, exacerbate old injuries, and make you more prone to new injuries. It is important to address these internal problems in order to reach optimal levels in fitness and in life.

AVOID BURNOUT

Burnout just might be the disease of the twenty-first century. Many people are imbalanced from being frequently exhausted, and struggle to shake the fatigue. A balanced life, a positive self-care routine, and good adrenal and hormonal health are all essential in preventing burnout. When you have adrenal fatigue, you may feel overly tired for no reason, be easily emotionally triggered, and be unable to sleep throughout the night. These few symptoms can have a large impact on your ability to exercise and stay committed to your health. In addition, if you exercise too much when your body is already overstressed, you can negatively impact your thyroid function. If you are diagnosed with adrenal fatigue, it's important to work with a holistic health practitioner to establish an individualized plan and ensure you are taking care of yourself.

BRAIN TRAINING

When you set the goal to become more active, it is common to train improperly and cause imbalances or injuries. Many athletes and other successful individuals have faced setbacks like physical injuries and concussions that they have had to overcome to advance. I experienced this myself. Due to head injuries and soft tissue injuries that had never healed properly, I experienced movement issues, dizziness, headaches, migraines, light sensitivity, nerve pain, chronic pain, cognitive issues, and mood issues. In my neurobiomechanical training with Z Health Education, I learned that these physical deficits and imbalances were decreasing my overall performance. Luckily, it is possible to improve our performance — including our strength, reaction time, flexibility, and ability to focus, read, and understand — and to decrease our pain through moving the body in specific and individualized motions catered to our injuries, including the eyes. Your eyes play a key role in how you move and how you perceive the environment around you. The eyes take in the information to feed to the brain - and pain is an output coming from the brain. The nerves and eyes send feedback to the brain, which then sends out a signal to tell your body if it is safe to move, how to move, or whether or not to feel pain. When we improve the information being fed to the brain, we can improve overall performance, decrease the perceived threat level in the body, improve your quality of life. In addition to working with the eyes and movement of the body in a safe way, it is also crucial to address the inner ear, nerve sensory pathways, and brain. In this way, we can reduce many of our symptoms and massively improve our well-being.

GET STARTED AND FEEL ALIVE

At one point in my life, it was excruciating to sit, to walk, to lie down. It was difficult to find words, to concentrate, to think, to be patient. I had constant emotional outbursts, my stomach hurt all the time, my digestion was horrible, eating didn't make me feel good, my sleep was off, lights and noise were threatening and over-stimulating, and I struggled to keep my mind positive. Let's be serious, it is hard to stay positive when everything around you is constantly makes you feel threatened. At the start of my journey to healing, I took one action daily, whether it was getting a massage, going for a walk, making homemade broth, taking supplements, getting rest, or doing visual drills / eye and vision exercises. I also moved daily, starting with ten minutes at a time. I didn't compare myself to what I once was but rather to how I was better than the day before, keeping in my mind what it would look and feel like to have attained my goal of perfect health.

I have also trained for a fitness competition, which entailed training two to three times a day, eating clean, making sleep a priority, and surrounding myself with other disciplined and determined individuals. Training for this competition was one of the best times of my life. I felt on top of my game and on top of the world: physically fit, mentally strong, and looking great. My confidence soared and I developed a strong positive self-image; I was doing what I said I would do even when I didn't feel like it, and I was getting amazing results. I willed myself to be my best and perform at my best and that determination required me to improve all areas of my life! I encourage you to challenge yourself and find what makes you feel most alive.

MINDSET AND ATTITUDE

To continue to advance and succeed when overcoming challenges or taking on a new one, mindset and attitude are key. Both play a crucial role in growth, whether it be exercising for the first time in your life, competing in a fitness competition, attaining good health, healing, or living a life you love. If you don't believe in yourself or in the attainment of your goals, then you will most likely not reach them. As Napoleon Hill said, "Whatever the mind of man can conceive and believe, it can achieve." Have a growth mindset, not a fixed mindset; a mindset of possibility and faith, not a mindset of victimhood and fear.

Many successful people first create their goal in their mind and then follow that vision in real life. Imagine yourself having reached your goal and then ask yourself what one thing you could do today to bring you closer to that vision. There are numerous ways to envision your dream life. Create a vision/goal board with pictures or words describing the goal you want to achieve. Keep a gratitude journal to train your brain to think in a gratitude mindset; like attracts like, so this will help you attract more to be grateful for. Write your goals down and carry them with you to look at throughout the day.

I recommend you begin by choosing one or two habits to change to help you reach your goals. You must be persistent and committed to changing these habits. Get clear on why you want to accomplish your goal and what positive impacts these habit changes can have on your life. See yourself as the person you wish to be, the person who has accomplished your goal already. Do not stop until you get there. When you reach it, set your next target. Soon you will look back and see the small changes you made and actions you took daily that led you to your big, hairy, audacious dream.

MIND HEALTH

Changing your life will require you to do something you haven't done before and to be someone who you haven't been before. To do this, you'll need to strengthen your will and develop the discipline to give yourself a command and follow through on it. Meditation can be very helpful in persisting despite perceived obstacles. This practice can improve your ability to be disciplined, to make the right habit changes, to stay positive, and to take action. Strengthening the power of my mind through meditation has improved my ability to have a clear, calm mind and to stay focused on my goals and the actions required to get me there instead of on the obstacles I face.

SELF-IMAGE

I know that self-image is a common struggle for many: the cycles of gain weight, lose weight, love yourself, sabotage yourself, and resent yourself. A positive self-image is still something I work on today, and I think it is something we will always have to consciously choose. It is essential to have a positive mindset and a positive self-image. When you develop a positive self-image, it will drive you to make healthy choices that align with your goals. You will eat to live, not live to eat. You will exercise to be healthy, not just to be skinny or as punishment for eating. You will eat clean because it allows you to enjoy life to the fullest, not because someone told you to. So choose to love yourself exactly as you are and exactly as you are not. There is only one of you, and the world needs you and your gifts. Choose healthy options because you choose to live a long, healthy life.

HOLISTIC HEALTH TO FREEDOM

Whether you are training for a fitness competition or just beginning your health journey, it is essential to pay attention to all three key factors: mindset, movement, and nutrition. Your performance and your health depend on it. I hope that my stories can inspire you to believe that no matter what you're going through, you are enough and you have everything you need to succeed. You, too, can heal. Just pick a place in your life and get started. You deserve to be the best you and to enjoy all that life has to offer. Stay happy and healthy through movement, a positive mindset, and good nutrition.

Find your Fitness to Freedom!

10

MY JOURNEY TO BECOMING A VIKING NINJA WARRIOR

"The strengths that define you are the reasons you will succeed in your journey. Move forward and blaze your own trail."

BY: NADIA DEDIC

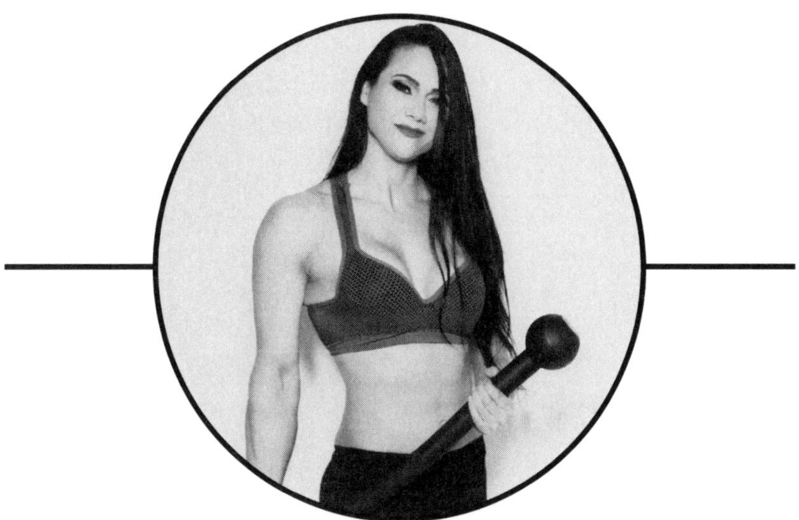

Nadia is a Certified Raw Foods Chef (CRFC) with the Raw Food Chef Alliance. She attended the Pachavega vegan culinary school specializing in raw food chef training and plant-based culinary arts. This distinct path led her to learn more about health and vitality and to implement a positive philosophy of living through the integration of a healthy diet and lifestyle. Nadia is currently enrolled in the Precision Nutrition Level 1 Program, which is home to some of the world's top nutrition coaches. With this training, she hopes to motivate and empower others to live a healthy and vibrant life.

Nadia obtained her Viking Ninja's Mindfulness Mechanics and Steel Mace Yoga Level 1 certification through Erik Melland, the Onnit Gym Steel Mace Master Coach and trainer to UFC Champions, and Erin Furry, Viking Ninja Master. Nadia also has her Paddle into Fitness Stand-up Paddle (SUP), SUP Yoga, and SUP Fitness certifications and received her Level 1 WPA (World Paddle Association) Certificate in 2019. Nadia is a believer in the mind's power and its ability to exceed perceived limits and hopes to encourage and support others in their own journey to health and wellness.

https://rawfoodchefalliance.com/certified-chefs

ig: @nd_squared

dedicatedliving.com

At any given time, an ordinary moment can become the catalyst to an extraordinary event, a shift in perspective that may take you on an unexpected journey. A simple conversation can spark an idea or reignite a passion. An opportunity can arise to work on a project you never dreamed was possible. A date can lead to a lifelong relationship or friendship. Even an unexpected hardship, illness, or tragedy could present an opportunity for great change. All these events have the potential to create a profound effect that could redirect your life's path at any given moment. As we have all learned in our own capacity, life has a way of creating its own agenda.

THE ACCIDENT

Like most people who live in the city, I dreaded the daily commute to the office. I had always led an active lifestyle, so I decided that cycling to the office was a better alternative than taking any form of transit. I enjoyed the independence cycling afforded me and how it transformed my daily commute into a form of therapy amid the rigors of working life. The freedom it provided was invaluable.

Despite vast improvements in cycling infrastructure in many cities, there is always a risk that when you pull those two wheels off the bike rack, you could succumb to some misfortune. One fateful morning, I was riding in the bike lane, with the wind in my hair and a false sense of security, when a vehicle struck me as I passed through an intersection. The driver made a right turn without signaling and lost sight of me during the turn. My leg twisted around more than one hundred and eighty degrees. The driver didn't realize he had hit me, and the car dragged me about twenty feet before he was flagged down by onlooking pedestrians. The result was a multitude of injuries, several surgeries, and an ongoing battle of rehabilitation and therapy. My only recollection from the accident was the gratitude I felt for the empathetic individuals who took immediate action to rush to my assistance.

THE AFTERMATH

Along with my physical injuries, I began to suffer mentally and emotionally after the accident and developed clinical depression. It was a feeling I had never had to endure before, and one that is indescribable to someone who has never had to experience or deal with depression. I cannot articulate it in words. Depression unfolds in different ways and can take on different shapes and forms depending on its power and complexity at any given moment. Triggered at the least expected times and tough to tackle by even the strongest of minds, depression can take a hold of you when you least expect it.

Anyone who has suffered a debilitating accident or injury can attest to the struggle and hardships that these circumstances create. In addition to the mental and physical battles, what I did not expect was the loss of my identity and independence. At the time, I managed and played women's premier soccer for the city of Toronto, I was an avid hiker who tackled sections of the Bruce Trail, and I connected to my community through competitive sport or team training. After the accident, I momentarily lost purpose in my life, and it would be a long, arduous battle to get back to "normalcy."

As the self-doubt compounded in my mind, I started to ask myself... If I was so competent in all other areas in my life, then why was I allowing these struggles to persist, despite my strong desire to change them? I recognized that finding the wisdom inside the hardships is one of the most valuable life lessons. Sometimes you just have to let yourself go and brace for the unknown. If I continued to view myself as a victim of circumstance, which is how I spent most of my time during those days, I would never be able to lift myself back up. I made the conscious decision to change my perspective and redirect my energy. How was I able to do this and how can you use this information to navigate through your own hardships? Let me show you.

MEANING THROUGH HARDSHIP

As Steven Hayes alludes to in his book, *Get Out of Your Mind and Into Your Life*, I was spending a lot of energy struggling with my pain but not getting much out of the struggle in terms of empowerment. Hayes states that "letting go of control does not require a lot of effort but letting go of control is tricky. It is confusing. And it is frustrating."[1]

Part of the human experience is the remarkable ability to move ahead even when faced with the most difficult of circumstances. With this in mind, I endeavored to let go of control and instead to seek meaning in my situation. I began to realize that I had an opportunity to reinvent myself and I started to change the questions I was asking in order to get different results. What would I need to do in this moment to capitalize on these unfortunate events? How could I develop the fortitude and resilience to move forward and become a better version of myself? How could I let go of control to free up and redirect my energy? At this time, acceptance and commitment became two of the most powerful tools in my arsenal to begin the healing process.

LEARNING HOW TO MANAGE YOUR STATE OF MIND

We cannot escape pain, difficulty, failure, injury, or heartache. Despite our best efforts to protect ourselves, at some point we are all subject to suffering in one form or another. We need to somehow get back up and move forward.[2] But how do we do that effectively when we don't have the energy to do so?

Through asking these challenging questions, I learned that how I chose to feel in any given moment was in fact completely within my

[1] Hayes, Steven C. and Smith, Spencer. 2005. *Get Out of your Mind and Into Your Life.* Oakland, CA: New Harbinger Publications.

[2] Pagliarini, Robert. (2011, August 25). Become Unbreakable: 10 Tips to Create More Personal Resilience. Retrieved from https://www.pickthebrain.com/blog/become-unbreakable-10-tips-to-create-more-personal-resilience/

control. If I could control my thoughts, I could directly impact my energy. For me, regaining control meant getting back to the basics and developing a plan to get back on track.

I've done a lot of reading over the years, and one thing I have learned is that in order for a plan to be successful, you need to define your *why*. Once you have that defined, you can set your short-term and long-term objectives to help you stay on track. Once your objectives are set in place, break down each goal into what you need to do monthly, weekly, and daily to keep the momentum going. Having a solid plan to move forward gave me the inner strength and motivation to better manage my state of mind and help me stay focused when I came up against unexpected setbacks or challenges.

I researched how to optimally recover from the accident through diet and functional strength training and sought to understand the balance between learning, mentoring, and action. As a result, I defined and implemented the following goals and objectives:

1. reintroduced training and sports back into my life in a balanced and efficient way;
2. developed a healthy, plant-based diet to help advance and support my body and mind during the recovery process;
3. built, and consistently engaged in a support system that I could reach out to when I needed help;
4. enlisted the help of leaders, mentors, and role models who could offer insight, research, and crucial lessons for me to excel and move forward.

BECOMING A CERTIFIED RAW FOOD CHEF

In March 2018, I embarked on a journey to explore the health benefits of following a plant-based diet, more specifically converting to a raw vegan diet for a period of time to see how it would impact me. After a recommendation from a friend, I attended the Pachavega vegan culinary school facilitated by Danielle Arsenault for a two-week retreat in Nicaragua. Through this program, I obtained my Raw Foods Chef Certification (CRFC) and became part of the Raw Food

Chef Alliance. My goal in attending the program was to learn how to deal with pain management and inflammation naturally through diet and nutrition.

This program taught me how proper nutrition can influence not only your physicality but your emotional state as well when planned and properly executed. It helped me become a raw food chef expert and accelerate my healing through raw food nutrition. I learned the nutritional benefits of whole foods and how they can support total body wellness. Eating in this manner includes, but is not limited to, fresh organic raw fruits and vegetables, nuts, fermented foods, sprouted foods, foods that are not heated above temperatures of around one hundred and fifteen degrees Fahrenheit (typically through the use of a dehydrator), and no processed or refined products.

I learned various technical skills in the kitchen and practiced everything I needed to know to be fully independent and creative in this new food journey. The program helped me heal emotionally, and I noticed the following physical benefits almost immediately:

- My joint inflammation subsided.
- My digestion improved because the food I was eating was rich in nutrients and enzymes.
- I had more energy, an increased vitality, and a more positive outlook on life.

I lost weight because the fiber in the raw fruits and vegetables kept me feeling satiated, enabling me to make healthier eating decisions throughout the day.

This experience led me on a distinct path to learning more about health and vitality, and toward implementing a positive philosophy of living from the heart through integrating a healthy diet and lifestyle. These changes empowered me to make other improvements in my life, and I was now ready to start the next phase in my recovery: strength through exercise and endurance, both mentally and physically. Ann Wigmore once said, "Your health is what you make of it. Everything you do and think either adds to the vitality, energy, or spirit that you possess or takes away from it."

FUNCTIONAL STRENGTH TRAINING: VIKING NINJA WARRIOR

In the book *Motivate Yourself and Reach your Goals*, Francis Coombes states that "to succeed you have to take risks that take you away from your comfort zone and push you beyond your boundaries . . . Use your senses – they will give you immediate feedback."[3] This quote resonated with me and helped me understand that to excel in life, you need to be open to the discomfort of the unknown and take advantage of the opportunities that present themselves whenever possible. Don't allow your self-doubt to creep in and limit your potential. I had spent too much of my life letting my fears interfere with my self-growth, and I wasn't about to let that continue any longer.

Erik Melland, Onnit Gym Steel Mace Master Coach and trainer to UFC Champions, and Erin Furry, Viking Ninja Master, brought the Viking Ninja Training System Workshop to Toronto, Canada for the first time. The steel mace is one of the few tools that can build muscle, improve anatomical function, and increase nervous system activity while training. What I learned from the workshop was how to use a steel mace to smoothly transition from one movement to the next in a continuous sequence through multiple planes of motion. I was introduced to this workshop through Adam Lecker, a functional training specialist. I was having difficulty with conventional training as it seemed to stress my body and aggravate my injuries. I had never heard of steel mace training before, but I was willing to try anything. What I came to learn was that the steel mace is one of the most effective tools with which to train and condition your whole body while mimicking real life movement. Mace training incorporates agility, balance and coordination and makes me feel empowered. And so it began . . . my journey to becoming a Viking Ninja Warrior.

I received the Viking Ninja's Mindfulness Mechanics and Steel Mace Yoga Level 1 certification, and I continue to practice and excel in this sport. I don't compare my progress to others; rather, I focus on doing what is best for my body. Fitness is about balance and developing a healthier relationship with yourself and your body to improve

[3] Coombes, Francis. 2013. *Motivate Yourself and Reach Your Goals.* Abington, UK: Teach Yourself.

your mental and physical health. There are no greater feelings than finishing a workout and knowing you gave it everything you have and drawing inspiration from those around you working hard toward their own objectives. No one said it's easy, and sometimes it's harder than you ever expected, but it's always worth the effort.

HOW TO OVERCOME OBSTACLES AND PERSEVERE

Life lessons are full of wisdom because they often have to be learned the hard way. There will be days of triumph and satisfaction, and others that will challenge you and create doubt in your mind about your capabilities. These are the moments that you need to remind yourself that any positive act or habit that you can carry out today is an action of who YOU will be tomorrow. Do not underestimate the power of daily habits as your habits determine who you ultimately become. Go back to your plan, revisit, reassess, and get focussed. Learn to adopt positive self-talk and measure your successes.

Start a gratitude journal or a develop a mantra that will keep you grounded and grateful. Take the time to reassure yourself that you are worth the effort; that will go a long way in helping you achieve your goals. Make sure you are establishing realistic goals, being flexible when required, and reaching out to your support system. Controlling and challenging the story you tell yourself daily will be your greatest weapon of success, along with gratitude and grace.

THE UNEXPECTED OUTCOME

Along this journey of life, we are offered a series of initiations, triumphs, and hardships as a means to challenge us to become a better version of ourselves and gain a better understanding of our purpose. A fundamental change in perspective shifted how I was able to interpret and deal with my traumatic circumstances. The lesson I took away from my experience, which I implore you to consider when faced with your own hardships and challenges, is that we can make radical progress toward our goals if we surround ourselves with the right support system and just put one foot in front of the other. On the other side of struggle is emotional and physical independence and empowerment. Fitness to Freedom and beyond.

11

SUPER MODEL, SUPER MOM

"You can do ANYTHING when you believe you can"

BY: SHARLENE ROCHARD

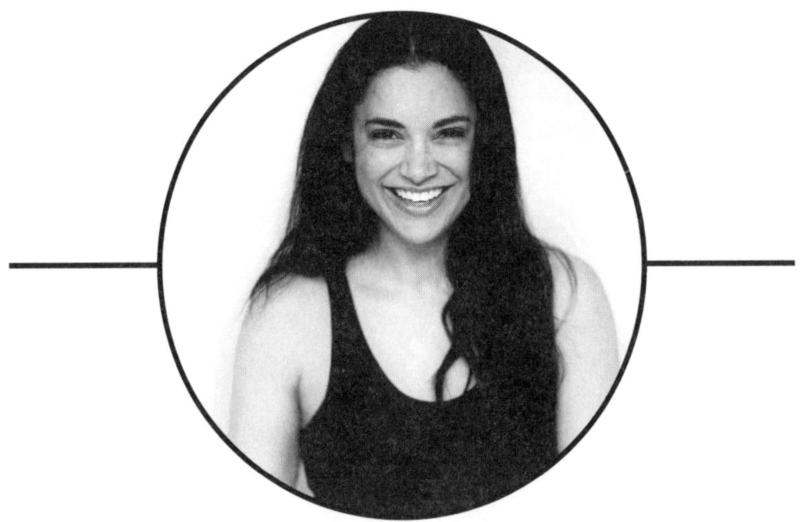

Sharlene Rochard was born in Ontario, Canada to parents of Trinidadian and European descent. Sharlene knew exactly where she was going in life from a very early age. At the age of four, she started performing in theater productions. At age thirteen, she became Miss Pre-Teen Canada.

The launch of her professional modeling career soon followed. Sharlene became one of the most successful and sought-after models in Canada, featured in many campaigns and major magazines. By age seventeen, she had traveled the world as a model.

Sharlene's exotic looks and diversity booked her nationwide TV commercials and music videos.

After studying acting at The Neighborhood Playhouse in New York and The Beverly Hills Playhouse in Los Angeles, she landed her first movie: The Little Richard Story, directed by Robert Townsend. She has grown her filmography ever since.

Sharlene was born to perform and has been in the public eye since she was four. Her life has taught her many things, including how to stay in shape. She takes care of everything in her life from her career and her body to her four children. Sharlene enjoys cooking, gardening, and everything fitness.

www.sharlenerochard.com

ig: @sharlenerochardlund | fb: @SharleneRochard

"If you think you can, you can." This mantra, which has been passed down from my grandmother to my mother to me and my children, is ingrained deep within my unconscious. I now pass it on to you, reader. This is a story of how to get tough when the tough get going, how to never let your inner self compete with your outer self, and how to rise above and realize that you are worth every single moment the universe has in store for you.

Growing up, I had no self-confidence. I was that klutzy kid who stared at my feet so I did not have to look anyone in the eye for fear they would poke fun of me. Grace, style, and fitting in with the crowd did not come easily to me. One day, my mother decided to enroll me in finishing school. This school entered their students in a modeling contest every year — and I won! Miss Klutz who never fit in anywhere won! After this contest, I entered the world of modeling and never looked back. The girl who had no confidence learned how to fake it, hold it all in (meaning suck in your stomach), hold her head up high, and step into the uncompromising world of fashion.

I became an international model who traveled the world. All those kids who hated me eventually learned of my success, and some even apologized for spitting on me on the school playground. I accepted their apology because they had taught me how to deal with the scrutinizing world of modeling. Everything serves a purpose, even the mean kids on the playground. I felt ready to conquer the world. I was featured on countless magazine covers and in commercials, music videos, and movies. I had found where I belonged and still belong to this day.

However, my life came to a screeching halt when I became pregnant with twins. Twelve weeks into the pregnancy, I went into pre-term labor. At the hospital, my doctor told me, "You are going to stay the duration of your pregnancy. You have a short cervix and three growing fibroids. If you leave this hospital, you will lose those babies."

I was petrified. I did not know what to do, but then my mantra pushed into overdrive: *If you think you can, you can.* I made the decision to have these babies and began to pray. During the prayer, two angels came to me. I could not see their faces, but they said, "You and your babies are going to be okay." I did not tell anyone what I had seen, but I told the doctor I would stay in the hospital and have these children no matter what it took.

A few days later, I had a cerclage surgery to tie my cervix together. I stayed in the Trendelenburg position for the rest of my pregnancy, which means lying down with your head below your waist. The weight of the growing fibroids and babies was too much for my short cervix, so I was not allowed to get up. I ate, slept, and spent five and a half months in that position. I still hold the record for the longest stay in the hospital and the earliest admitted pregnancy.

Twelve weeks is very early, and if we had been anywhere else in the world with any other doctor, they would have just let me miscarry. However, my doctor is one of the best high-risk pregnancy doctors in the world. This was not a coincidence. As I lay there day after day, I was called upon to help other women who were also told they could not leave until they deliver. I mentored these women and told them my story. They gained confidence in themselves and would often say, "If she can do it, so can I." I became an inspiration to the other women on the floor as I told them my mantra.

On June 11, it was time to deliver the miracle babies. They were healthy but needed to stay in the NICU. These two souls had chosen me to be their mother. I had worked hard to get them into this world, but I had no idea how to raise them or even give them a bath! I learned quickly, as every mother does, but this new job was the hardest I have ever taken on.

After being in the hospital for so long, I had developed hospital depression, postpartum depression, and muscle atrophy; on top of it all, I had twins, which meant no sleep. There is a reason that moms of multiples need support.

Just seven months later, I was pregnant again. I had gone from being a top model booking every job to being stuck in the hospital pregnant with twins to being pregnant again. Another angel came to me, this time in the form of a woman who guided me through the tough feelings surrounding getting pregnant again so quickly. I had another cerclage and Olivia was born a healthy, happy baby.

Now this fitness model had three children all under the age of two. My body was destroyed. I had not fully recovered from muscle atrophy and depression, and I found three babies almost impossible to care for. But I kept my mantra: *If you think you can, you can.* I kept it together for fourteen months — until I became pregnant again. This was not supposed to happen! I was determined not to have this baby and decided to go to the women's clinic to take the abortion pill. I was just beginning to lose the weight after two pregnancies, and I did not feel like my body could do it one more time.

The night before I was scheduled to go to the clinic, another angel came to me. He said, "Mommy, why don't you want me? I am a good boy."

In the morning, I told my husband what had happened. He said, "If it is a boy and if what you are saying is true, we have to keep the baby." I canceled my appointment and waited for a gender test. It was a boy. The angel was real. We were going to do this again.

If I think I can, I can, and I did! I had four kids in three and a half years. I dealt with severe depression and anxiety, became a mother four times, and to top it all off, lost my father. My life as I once knew it had completely shattered. After being in such a self-conscious business since the age of twelve, my outer beauty was all I had until I was forced to use my mind and overcome obstacles that the universe knew I could handle. Life can beat you up at times.

How did I go through all of this and come out believing that whatever life throws at you, you can throw right back a thousand times harder? How did I take care of four children all under the age of four and keep my sanity? How did I lose the weight and keep it off so I can continue my quest to inspire women with the knowledge that your mind, not your body, defines you\? I want to tell you how I freed myself from the shackles that limited me and help you find your own mantra to free yourself so you can lose the weight and love your body for all that it can do.

My life was full of outside opinions, but I realized that all other people do is hold up a mirror and show us the relationship we have with ourselves. In order to deal with life, you need to organize your own thoughts and put other people's opinions in a box on the shelf. Every other relationship you have comes second to the relationship you have with yourself. In order to move past all of my disempowering thoughts — *I can't; these kids are driving me crazy; my life sucks; how did I get here?; I was a supermodel, and now I am just a mom; I can't believe my life; where did the time go?* — I needed to create a new me. I dreamed of what I wanted to be and asked myself, "Do I want to be fit, in shape, eating well, and loving life?" The answer was YES! So I created that new horizon for myself.

Take a moment and clear your mind. Where are you in life right now? What do you deserve? Where do you want to be in one year, five years, ten years? Write it all down. Grab a journal and honestly look at yourself right now. Break the barriers of self-limitation.

The next step is to analyze what you wrote. Look at all the negative beliefs you have and change the words into positive affirmations. For example, I would often say, "I hate my body. My kids ruined my body. I can't go back to modeling looking like this; nobody wants a model who has four kids and stretch marks." I changed those words into "I only get one body, so I need to take care of myself. The kids made me realize the strength I hold within."

I had four lives who depended on me, and now I was going to get my own life back. Life comes in waves; periods of stillness can evolve into large changes if the wind is blowing in the right direction. It is up to you create your self-worth and self-esteem. Make your waves count.

People have sixty thousand thoughts a day, but we often think the same thoughts over and over. Imagine what your life would be like if you only concentrated on the good thoughts. In addition to "If I think I can, I can," I use several other mantras as well:

I am constantly increasing my wealth

I am constantly increasing my love for myself

I am successful

I can and will prosper

Even though I had worked to change my mind, I still had bad habits, such as not drinking enough water, binge eating, and eating my kids' unfinished meals. My mindset was positive, but now I had to get my body back on track. Humans are creatures of habit. Once a person sticks to a new routine for twenty-one days, it becomes the new normal. I kept a journal of everything I was eating and how I felt as I ate it. It is important to notice what, when, and why you are eating. One thing I noticed through my food journal was that whenever my kids were playing loudly and I was reaching my boiling point, I would turn to candy.

I was not alone. People often turn to sweets when they are feeling stressed. Any form of carbohydrate triggers the brain to make serotonin, that feel-good chemical that can help take the edge off of anger, frustration, and other feelings of anxiety that overwhelm us. Sugar digests faster than slower burning carbohydrates so the feel-good response happens faster. But sleep also replenishes our serotonin. Getting enough sleep is important because if you are sleep-deprived, your body tries to get energy and that feel-good boost from food, making the urge to binge eat very strong. Not getting enough sleep also starts to raise cortisol levels, causing the body to store fat. The term "getting my beauty sleep" are words of truth.

The strongest muscle in the body is not the heart: it is the tongue. Speak positive thoughts and eat foods that are healthy. I chose to eat a plant-based diet that ideally emphasizes raw or lightly steamed vegetables, fruits, whole grains, legumes, and occasionally a small piece of meat or fish. I also eat a lot of foods that aid in weight loss. Grapefruit contains health-promoting phytochemicals such as lycopene, beta-carotene, limonin, naringenin, and the antioxidant vitamin C. All these ingredients are amazing for our health. They aid in weight loss and cellulite reduction, boost immunity, fight diseases like cancer, and benefit your skin. I also include blueberries, ginger, cucumbers, eggs, lemons, and all greens in my diet. Consuming eggs, oatmeal, ginger, garlic, chili powder, and greens can also aid in the thermic effect. Thermic Effect increases your metabolism by food processing, and promotes how the body stores the food digested.

Drinking water also helps with weight loss. If you are even moderately dehydrated, your metabolism slows down by three percent. That could mean on average fifty calories a day added without you even knowing it. Those extra calories could be just the stubborn five pounds you want to lose! Water also carries nutrients and oxygen, aids in digestion, promotes healthy blood, and rids the body of excess toxins. I carry a water bottle everywhere I go and drink as much water as I can daily.

The next step is exercise. After having four children in three and a half years and rehabilitating through muscle atrophy, I struggled to get back into shape. I started slowly, worked up my endurance, and began building muscle. Getting in shape is easier when the whole family is involved. I never understood why parents sit and watch their children play on the playground. I do pull-ups, squats, jumping jacks, and other exercises using the playground equipment. Parents who are active tend to have active kids. Kids are always watching.

I am grateful for all of my children and for everything life has thrown at me because I believe we are all here on this earth to learn. Getting in shape is mostly mind over matter. If you believe you can, you can. Live the life you want right now. Make the change in your mindset and a healthy lifestyle will become second nature. Be positive and use uplifting mantras as you take the steps to create what you want, and you will achieve success.

If you think you can, you can!

12

MONSOON

"When the worst, most impossible scenario falls upon us, we may fall and spiral down into our sorrow and misery. Or we may choose to get up and let all ruins become a reason to triumph."

BY: RACHEL BALUNSAT

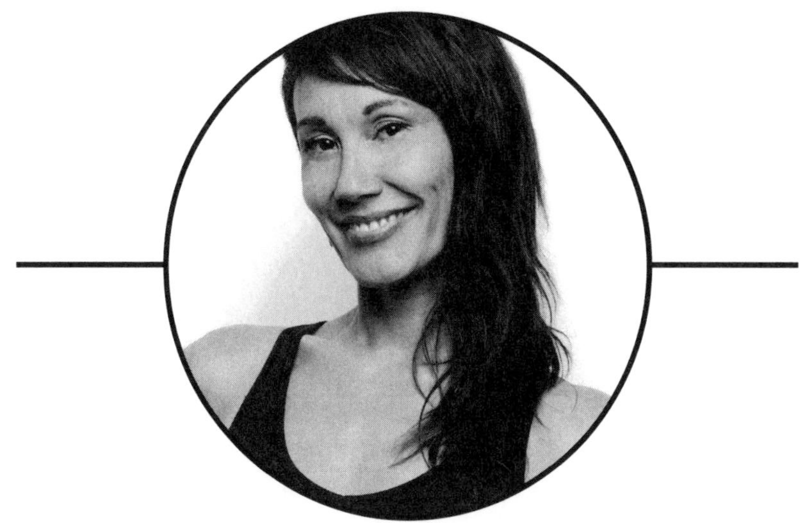

Born and raised in San Francisco by an American mother and Filipino father, Rachel Balunsat was given a unique bicultural perspective of the world. Her studies lead her to sociology and psychology. Then, while living in Spain during college, art classes revealed a new direction. Rachel became an award winning wedding photojournalist traveling the world for over a decade. However after having a challenging bout with health for many years she became an Ayurvedic health practitioner eventually healing herself with plant based nutrition. Now Rachel competes as a vegan bodybuilder and has won several competitions in her mid forties. Her pastimes include visionary painting, gardening and yoga, all of which she sees as her part in creating a sustainable world. Currently Rachel is working on a memoir.

ig: @wildess_superfoods_alchemist

fb: @rachel.balunsat

On Sept 8th, 2014 I received an unforgettable phone call. One that every human being dreads, yet anticipates, and still hopes will never happen. The afternoon sun illuminated a hot hazy light. Vast quiet soared over dry grassy knolls and the ancient knobby oak trees of Sonoma County. I had just settled in, decorated my new home, and found myself able to breathe in the great, warm, expansive view of the mountains from my deck. Steve, my dear stepfather, friend and man who raised me out of my twenties, asked me through the airwaves from several states away, "Rachel, Can you sit down please?" I remembered my mother explaining why we sit down to hear bad news... We might faint. She told me that when she was twenty-one she received a phone call that her father had died in a tractor accident. She screamed at the top of her lungs and could not stop screaming. I sat down in my low Balinese wicker meditation chair. I breathed in. I breathed out...

"Your mother is missing."

"What do you mean, Steve?"

"We were driving your mom to her doctor's appointment," he continued, "We tried to drive through a flash flood but it pulled us out into the wash ..." My ear hung on his words, dismayed and desperate for details to clarify. My stepfather paused, "The medics are looking for her in a helicopter... I'm so sorry Rachel. I'm so sorry."

When I was a little girl, I used to cry because I could not fathom the idea of my mother dying. I would look up into her big almond brown eyes, two deep pools of love cushioned by her long curled eyelashes, and I would often cry for how much I loved her. Her soft wavy auburn hair framed her beautiful square German jaw. Steve once admired that she had the face of a movie star. My mother would tell me as she held me against her bosom, "Sweetheart, I am not going to die for a long, long, long, long time. By the time that happens you will have a family of your own, and you will have the love of everyone around you. It will be so much easier to accept."

"Steve! Was she in the car???"

Steve relayed how they had been driving in the monsoon rushing to get to a doctors appointment. He had crossed the same stream in the road earlier and though he hesitated this time, unable to assess the current depth, he attempted to cross again. A flash flood of water yanked their car into the wash, a river of fast moving trees and debris.

I could barely breathe expecting the next moment. I asked for more and more detail. I wanted to know everything. *"Where is she Steve?? Is she in the car? Missing under the water somewhere?"*

When horror is described there is no end to the imagination. I had to know *exactly* in order to spare myself the pain of what was in my mind, visualizing my mother drowning in the car. He explained that he was able to swim to her side of the car as it was filling with water, and pry her door open against the gushing flood. He was able to get her out of her seatbelt and safely out of the car. They clung to the vehicle against the torrent, but she was swept out of his hands and into the rays of light that peaked through the Catalina Mountains. He had eventually swum to safety but barely made it out alive. There was now a helicopter looking for my mother.

I don't know that either of us had much hope. In some unspoken way we didn't dare hope because good news would rather surprise us than bad. I eagerly got off the phone to call my spiritual teacher. She was known for helping to find missing people with her deep clairvoyance; I trusted her ability to help in ways deeper than the ordinary. I got a hold of one of the monastics, who passed along the message. In the living room I sat carefully in front of my large altar on the sheepskin rug with my Tibetan singing bowl. The Buddha above held my steadiness as I dropped into meditation. The longest two hours of my life passed. I remained as calm as possible, opening up the interior of my heart and mind to the magic of the Universe and to the possibility of a miracle.

Emptiness. I disappeared into another world. Another realm. I wanted to hope and it terrified me. I prayed but didn't know what to pray for. If I prayed for life, death could devastate me. If I prayed for her peace in death I was abandoning her life. Would I then be responsible if she didn't make it? *How powerful is the mind?* I gathered myself in front of my altar and did the only thing I knew. I reached out through my meditations to all the highest realms of the Universe, to the highest angels, Jesus, Buddha, to every beautiful understanding I had ever known. I made my great appeal to the deep compassion of the Great Ones. I allowed every bit of energy in my being to be available to my mother. To ease any fear and bring her to safety whether in life or in death.

Months prior I had returned to the mainland from Kauai, to care for my ailing father in Pacifica. He was slowly dying of diabetes like his seven brothers and sisters had before him. At this point he had third stage kidney failure. On his eightieth birthday I had a party for him and he made several kinds of pancit: A thin, Asian rice noodle dish loaded with all the Filipino favorites; garlic and shiitakes, shrimp and scallions. I remember kneeling on the floor with my head in his lap. With tears in my eyes I looked up at him. I knew this might be the last time I would celebrate his birthday with him. He read my face and smiled. "I love you, Daddy." Tears dropped. We spent a lot of time talking about his death. Wondering about it. It was a topic that my father was very comfortable with. He felt both a warmth and an invitation towards it.

He and my mother were still friends and talked for hours sometimes. My mother gave me advice on how to care for my dad. My dad spoke fondly of my mother; How she was the love of his life, and the most intelligent, funny, and artful story teller. She was one of the most loving women I knew, doting on children everywhere. My best friend throughout life. My confidante, my cheerleader, my support. She reminded me of what amazing things were in store for me at all times in my life. She was the sun on the darkest of my days.

News came. My teacher contacted me, she had gone into meditation to find my mother.

"I am sorry to tell you this dear, but I think your mother didn't make it."

My stepfather called shortly after, "Rachel," he said, fragile with the deepest sadness and concern in his voice. I wanted to protect him from having to deliver this message to me. I knew it would devastate him.

"Your mother was found, she didn't make it. . . . I'm so sorry, I'm so sorry." I wanted to hold him. Tell him it was okay.

"I know," I said to him. "Rinpoche told me . . . I love you Steve." I remember little else. I continued on in my meditation as the world spiraled around me. A huge moon appeared in the sky that evening affirming some kind of inexplicable order to things. It became a symbol that held me and comforted me through the months and waves of grief. My mother's closest relative, cousin Sue, called me during a spiritual teaching I went to that night, "Rachel, are you okay? Do you need to talk? I am here for you." My mom's cousin Sue looked like my mom. She helped me imagine my mother, being like her sister with her matching brown eyes and wavy hair. That defining square jawline that had transferred to all of us cousins.

Between moments of peace there were moments of chaos with a series of unexpected endings. A few months later I was devastated by the ending of a long term relationship. I grasped everywhere for direction, purpose, meaning. I couldn't sleep, waking each morning to the emptiness of a blank future. I howled at unexpected moments in a relentless pain. Every kind of love left a vacancy. I was partnerless, I was motherless, I would be fatherless soon, and as a woman in my forties I felt I had missed any opportunity to have children. I felt there was no longer even a *purpose* to bear children. My motivation had always been to bring my mother's lineage through my offspring to further *her* legacy. I had only wanted to experience the bonding of grandmother and baby and relate to motherhood. I had wanted to be alongside my mother raising my child.

Mornings got earlier and earlier as I awoke to the train wreck of reality. I would pound away at the piano to resolve the morning pain. My sweet roommate, Michael, would sleepily shout to me, muffled through his pillow, "It sounds GREAT Rachel!" He was my rock. He tolerated me banging out my daily passions at 6am until I eventually became one of those unfathomable early morning gym goers. I needed to do something with myself in the mornings. I wouldn't drown in grief. No, I would become fit for the first time in my life. My mother would want me to continue to do great things. To be healthy, free, and alive. In my deep sadness and resentment towards my ex, I decided I would just BE the best I could be in spite of him. Damned if I would let myself be buried in self pity. I had always hated the gym, but it would become a familiar place available to me in my weirdest hours of wakefulness.

I did not understand what I was doing nor did I have any concept of a routine or form. Until one early morning I ran into a familiar, older, red headed gentleman with two long braids. He was a Hari Krishna. He was vegetarian, committed to meditation, simplicity and kindness. I asked him to tell me stories about Krishna to occupy my mind while I worked out. I found refuge in these sacred ancient tales. Like Christian parables of truth they delivered messages of how to be a good person in this world. And soon this monk-like, sports-geared man wearing a tennis-hat and two sweatbands on either wrist became known to me as Krishna Nick. I told him everything and quickly found a home in his compassion. Likewise, he found a home in my friendship. My mind was difficult to be alone with. Thankfully he followed me through my routine, gave me tips and showed me how to use the machines until I began to know my way around. I gained confidence and soon felt this was my second home.

Eventually in the same month as my mother passed, one year later, my father was on the brink of dying. Hospice had come and we were waiting for the end. I cherished each last minute. I remember my father's quandary: "How do I die, Rachel? How does it happen? I keep waiting. Am I gonna die? Or, am I gonna live?" It never occurred to me how elusive death itself could be at the moment we are waiting for its arrival. For my father it was like a long anticipated friend.

Shortly after he passed, I found myself living on the road traveling and eventually healing on a beautiful desert land that belonged to the owner of my company. I was taking his month long course in nutrition. My strength and stamina increased. I climbed crazy rocky mountains like a goat. I ran great distances where I received messages from the inspiring native land that imbued me with wisdom and words from my parents. Our community of health practitioners gathered each Saturday night at the large fire circle where we would share stories. The first Saturday night in the flickering silence under the stars, I shared the story of my mother's tragic death. The second Saturday I shared the story of my father's death and transformation. On the third Saturday, a friend got a hold of me at the Oasis to tell me that my recent roommate, my dear friend Michael who championed me on the piano as I grieved my mother, had shot himself in the head. I wailed as I departed back into the world's abyss. I bought a one way ticket to Oahu where I couch-surfed with compassionate friends I made and spent time with my feet in the ocean. It was there that I received the message that cousin Sue was dying quickly of lung cancer.

My world seemed to be collapsing as my circle of safety grew smaller and smaller, yet my health was rapidly improving, supporting my grief and giving me purpose. A team member suggested I get into competing. *Bodybuilding??* I never would have come up with that idea myself. You have got to be kidding. I could never look like that. I wasn't entirely sure I wanted to look like that. Of course, never being one to decline an opportunity, I joined Coach Frauka. A charismatic German knockout on a Harley, age fifty-six, and 1st place winner of many bodybuilding competitions. She cheered me and coached me into top performance over the course of three months. Then, two weeks before showtime, I received the news that a dear friend from college, one I'd been trying to reach, had died from an intestinal disorder. I binged on chocolate, felt like a failure, and was unable to help the people I loved. I lived in the irony of being a health practitioner unable to save my own friends and family. Yet I was determined not to give up. I didn't think I could do the competition. Frauka repeatedly called me as I avoided her and ignored her calls until I finally called back.

"Frauka, I don't think I can do it. I fucked up. I've been eating chocolate and junk for three days!" I was throwing in the towel.

The difference between a friend and a coach is that a friend would sympathize, empathize, give a person understanding and comfort. A coach holds out the finish line, points to what's possible without ever losing sight of the end goal.

"Rachel!" She spoke to me firmly, "JUST. GET. BACK. UP! Finish your binge, get back to the gym and do three extra cardio this week. You'll be fine!"

She had such enthusiasm, and such conviction that I began to believe her. Sometimes we borrow the faith of others when there is none left in ourselves. I moped for a couple more days until I was satisfied and then I miraculously pulled myself back to the gym. All I had to do was get my clothes on, get there and the rest would work itself out.

I binge watched competitions on YouTube, memorizing the winners' every movement. I noticed they didn't give a fuck about anyone else but their shining moment. And then I realized, I didn't give a fuck either. I went live on Facebook unboxing my sparkly, crystal, competition bikini telling the world what crazy shit I was up to. *I have nothing to lose* became my mantra. I had already lost everything. I really didn't care what anyone thought, including myself.

When I got backstage with all the sixpack, muscle armed women, they were all lifting weights to pump up. I found a pair of dumbbells and joined in. There was a comradery backstage I wasn't expecting. Women were boosting each other up with compliments, empowering each other to do great and be their best. I had never been around so many strong, fit, muscled up women. While I waited in line backstage in my platform heels and fuschia bikini, I dropped to the floor and did pushups; 10, 20, 30, 40! I kept going. We gobbled down rice cakes and honey. The starch and sugar was supposed to make the muscles pop. Life was good.

The evening gown masters was ages forty-plus. I glided out onto the stage and took 1st place. That felt like a cake walk. I wasn't impressed until I got to evening gown open, all ages competing. I strutted. I basqued in my five minutes of solo stage glory. I did whatever the hell I could think of to shine, gleam, radiate. I poured my heart out and looked up at God. This was MY moment. I gave thanks just to be on that friggin' stage with twenty-and-thirty-somethings somethings. And then, the judges called the top five back onto the stage...including myself. They announced fifth place, forth, then third. I began to sweat. My name hadn't been mentioned yet. Then second place was announced and again not my name. I was awestruck.

"And the first place winner is . . ."

I didn't even feel the trophy being pushed into my hands. I didn't know what I was doing or what I was supposed to do. I had just received my first place, pro card, at age forty-four in an all age category. I smiled and looked up at Frauka who ran up to me in tears.

"YOU DID IT!!"

HOW did I do it? I wanted to know! I held my two awards, one in each hand. I looked up to the sky and spoke into the great mystery of things.

"One for you mom," I said aloud. "And, one for you dad."

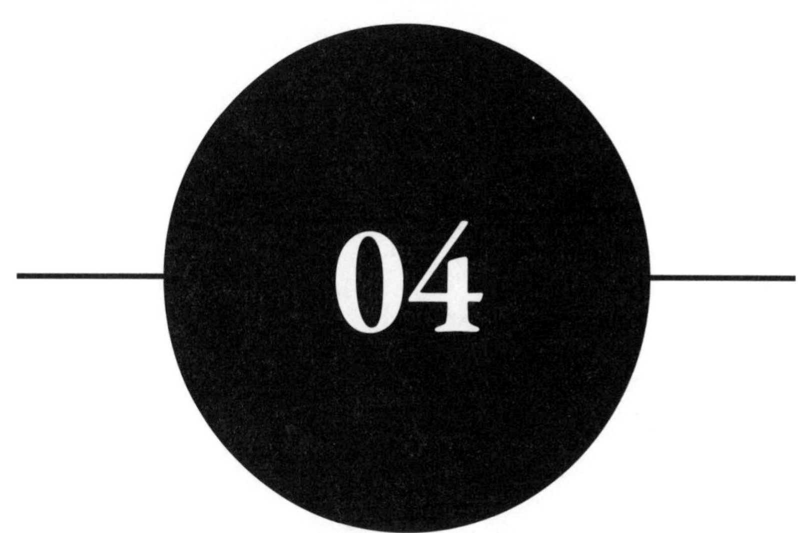

THE FREEDOM TO SELF-LOVE

13

UNDER THE SURFACE

"On the outside, I was the ultimate modern woman successfully managing all the roles in her life with ease and grace."

BY: TARRAH WYNN

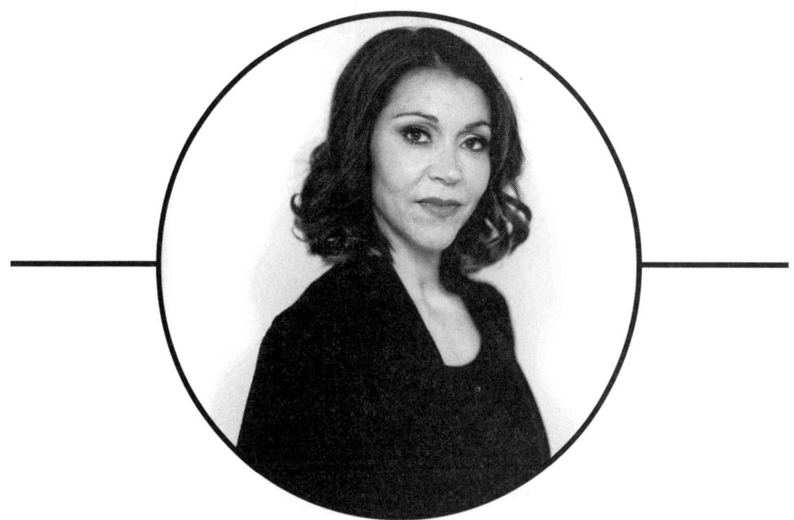

Tarrah was born and raised in a small town in Nova Scotia. She is a born leader and mentor who spent most of her career climbing the corporate ladder within the construction industry. Her formal education came in the form of a bachelor's degree with a major in history and a minor in sociology from Dalhousie University. Upon graduation, Tarrah enrolled in the Information Technology Institute where her love for business began to blossom.

Tarrah is a proud mother of two boys and a loving wife to her husband, Matt. Together they live in Southern Ontario. Tarrah has always had a passion for fitness and participated in various fitness competitions until at the age of thirty-seven, she found herself exhausted, inflamed, and no longer able to manage her fit physique. After rounds of tests, she realized that her strict eating regime, obsession with exercise, and workaholic mindset had caused this mom to burn out. With the realization of what she had done, Tarrah poured her heart and soul into learning how to heal her body with food, lifestyle, and mindset changes. A year later, she enrolled in the Institute for Integrative Nutrition where she studied to become a certified health coach. Today, Tarrah shares her story with other high-performing women who are struggling to manage it all. She has created a space in her business, Tarrah Wynn Holistic Health and Nutrition, where she teaches women how to balance their hormones, heal their gut, and reclaim their vitality.

I struggled for a long time to live a balanced life while juggling work, family, personal time, diet, and exercise. If I had a nickel for every time someone has said to me, "I don't know how you do it all!", I'd literally be rich. I suppose they mean it as a compliment, one designed to make women feel accomplished and powerful, evoking an image of Superwoman standing tall over her victims with sword in hand. Truth be told, though, that thought left me feeling distinctly uncomfortable and inadequate.

On the outside, I was the ultimate modern woman successfully managing all the roles in her life with ease and grace. I was the woman who could finish work on Friday, have a baby on Saturday, and not miss a beat. I was the woman who could take care of the house, the family, and the job and still stay fit and eat clean. This Superwoman, held back by nothing, appeared to have it all.

On the inside, though, I was gasping for air, struggling to stay afloat. My days compromised of doing all the things, checking off all the boxes, yet I was numb, exhausted, and feeling completely overwhelmed. I wanted the balance that everyone talked about but feared I did not understand how to get it. I was a slave to the gym and felt chained to the treadmill. I secretly wished I could be like those women who never worked out a day in their life and ate whatever they wanted, but I feared that if I stopped controlling things, everything would fall apart. Then the awful truth that I did not actually have it all together would be exposed.

How did I find myself facing such a dilemma? My life didn't start out this way. I did not think I was destined to be a powerhouse girl boss, a fitness competitor, or even a modern-day Superwoman — not even close. I began feeling like an outsider early, even though my parents raised me to believe I could be the first female Prime Minister if I wanted. During my childhood and into adolescence, I was so shy that I would break out in red welts all over my body when I had to speak in front of a group. *Did I fit in?* I certainly wasn't the very last person picked or the one the cool girls picked on, but I didn't excel at much. I was average at everything I tried. While my best friend made the varsity teams, aced the exams, and dated the cutest boys, there I was, not making the cut, getting B's and C's, and standing back at school dances. No matter how hard I tried, I felt like I was never as good as she. Best-selling author Brené Brown said it beautifully: "Sometimes the most dangerous thing for kids is the silence that allows them to construct their own stories — stories that almost always cast them as alone and unworthy of love and belonging." As my feelings of unworthiness grew in strength, my voice seemingly got weaker.

When I look back, I realize that those moments of not being athletic or extraordinarily smart in school were the very things that led me to find my love for fitness and my chance to shine as a solo competitor. From the moment I stepped into my first gym, I felt a deep sense of comfort and belonging. I didn't realize it then, but that gym, filled with sculpted bodies, smiling faces, and pure dedication, gave me a chance to prove that pure perseverance and hard work could overcome innate talent.

When I was twenty-one, a personal trainer at my gym noticed I had been making progress and suggested that I had the potential to do well in a bodybuilding competition. He agreed to train me for free, and much like a hungry puppy awaiting her next command, I followed suit. The mere fact that someone had seen my efforts led me to dive head-first into fourteen weeks of grueling workouts, two-a-day cardio sessions, and a restricted chicken, rice, and broccoli diet, no questions asked. I deeply desired to be noticed, to be discovered, and to live the life of the fitness models I envied so much. I believed this would be my chance to shine and have my place in the spotlight. Over the next eight years, I would train for three more competitions and professional photoshoots.

I have to admit, the attention I got when I was stage-ready felt amazing. People noticed me and commented on how great I looked. But weeks after the show, when the tan had disappeared and the body fat returned, the praise stopped. There it was, so ever-present: that little insecure voice in my head that perpetually reminded me I needed to try harder, have more discipline, and be leaner. This voice haunted me even when I stopped competing for good. For fitness competitors, it's hard to accept our body when we're not in peak condition; we feel fat, which only fuels the cycle of feeling inadequate.

I'll never forget the night after I won first place. In the lead-up to that competition, I was a few months into a new job, living with my then-boyfriend, and training night and day. My vision was clear, and I felt better during this preparation than I had for any competition before. My body was getting leaner and progressing ahead of schedule. I had blacked out one day during a posing practice with my coach, but I didn't care. My mind was focused: this time I would win.

My boyfriend had experienced many trials with depression throughout our relationship. I felt guilty for being so focused on myself during my contest preparation so I encouraged him to go out with friends and accept invitations from his colleagues. Well, that one backfired! Just weeks away from my show, I learned that he had been unfaithful with the work colleague whom I had encouraged him to spend time with.

There I was the night after my first-place win: homeless, single, and alone, sitting on my best friend's couch with a great set of abs covered in smelly fake tanning cream. I remember sitting there thinking, "This is it?" I was supposed to be at the after-party in a cute dress, eating and drinking and celebrating my win, not sitting there alone. All the years of sweat, dedication, and hard work — was it all for this?

Rarely when we're in the depths of life's most defining moments do we realize that this is where our true character is born. I would later learn that that moment was a pivotal point in my story, the point when I realized that being famous, getting discovered, and ultimately being worthy of belonging didn't come from six-pack abs or a plastic trophy. I would realize that my self-worth would not come until I was actually ready to receive it.

Although my realization that night began to give me a true sense of what I was capable of, I continued to struggle to balance food, workouts, and career over the next ten years. I had proven to myself that grit, hard work, and laser focus helped me survive, so I continued living life that way. I began to move up the corporate ladder quickly, bought my first home, got married, birthed two babies, and kept up the persona of a boss babe who had it all together. I was burning the candle at both ends.

And then came the fall. The harder I worked and the more restrictive I got, the more my body began to reject it all. I remember checking in with my coach one morning, terrified to send in my progress pictures. I would have to explain that I hadn't cheated, never missed a workout, and managed to get in all cardio sessions, yet I had gained weight. I was puffy and inflamed and my gut was a mess. I was drinking four cups of coffee and an energy drink every day but still struggling to stay awake during my morning drive to work. And no one knew. While I was doing everything I could, I still had a nagging feeling that maybe my efforts were just not enough. I carried on like this for another few months before deciding something bigger was wrong. I needed to get help.

As I began to search for answers, I came across a book promising a solution. I was desperate for anything to make me feel better, so I did the three-day detox it suggested. I can try to explain how it literally changed my life, but unless you've experienced pure mental clarity, it's hard to put into words. It felt like the fuzzy blanket that had been sitting on top of my brain had lifted, like the clouds had parted in the sky. A feeling of hope that I couldn't remember experiencing in so long emerged. That experience was the start of what felt like a rebirth. I became obsessed with learning everything I could about how to optimize my life through food. I began by seeking out a naturopath and every possible holistic healer I could find.

During that time, I had started a new job and had been feeling anxious and inadequate. I was afraid I had no business being in the position I was hired for. After achieving year after year in my former job, I suddenly felt like a beginner again. That little girl crept back in, telling me that I didn't deserve this new level of growth. Starting a new job is kind of like starting in a new high school where all the kids already know each other and have a secret language and their own way of doing things. I tried my best to learn what I didn't know, or at least what I thought I didn't know. The truth is, I really *did* know; I had just forgotten how to listen to my confidence.

Day after day, week after week, I peeled back the layers to rediscover who I was at the core. It felt like a combination of grief and ecstasy. I grieved because I had become numb to my emotions and had created a bubble of isolation around myself. I was sad that I had identified myself as a strong, professional, modern woman who would rather work than stay home with her kids, someone who would rather follow her meal plan than go out for dinner with friends. I knew that the earlier version of myself didn't know better at the time, but I was still sad for her and the experiences she missed out on. On the other hand, I felt ecstasy because the clues I received over the years, that little voice — they were confirmation that I could trust myself and know that the messages were there to show me the path I needed to follow. Now was the time to stop silencing them.

I became an obsessed student, lapping up every ounce of knowledge about health, natural healing, and self-development that I could. Yes, the girl who was never great at school, and especially not at science or math, geeked out over statistics, facts, and figures. As I began to understand how to nourish my body rather than punish it, my energy exploded, my brain fog disappeared, and my digestive issues vanished. I worked out for half my usual time doing workouts I loved and felt more fit and beautiful than I had in all my years performing in fitness competitions.

Perhaps it was the fear of not measuring up to those I admired, or maybe it was the fear of being seen for who I was and judged not good enough. Regardless, I had chosen to isolate myself from the outside world, particularly from other women. I believed that due to my leadership role at work, it would not be appropriate to forge relationships there. During my healing journey, I realized that I needed a community of like-minded, inspiring, and powerful women who felt like I did. I got extremely brave and joined communities where I knew no one. These connections allowed me to get vulnerable, share my stories, and develop deep emotional bonds that would change my old beliefs that women were competitive, needy, or untrustworthy. We tend to forget that humans are a social species, meant to belong to a group. Our genetic makeup makes us destined for community over disconnection.

Today when I get asked, "How do you do it all?", I politely and proudly say, "I don't!" I simply make it work and if that means that the laundry piles up or my hair isn't washed, so be it. Striving for an unrealistic image of perfection is not achievable, nor does it bring us a sense of having made it. I finally got it. I don't have to fit it all in. I don't have to strive to be someone other than who I am. When you let go of trying to do it all and make careful choices, you step into the driver's seat of your life. When you spend your time and energy on things that fill you up rather than drain you, life becomes much more satisfying. Your job, your family, and your life depend on you as the main ingredient, just as you are. If you haven't put your own oxygen mask on, you'll have little to offer others, no matter how much you want to. Claiming time for yourself and having the health you crave is not a luxury, and it will pay tenfold it you let it.

This life of ours is a journey that will take us down a winding, often rocky road, and it will not be perfect. Perfectionism is the belief that something has to be perfect to be enough. It's all-or-nothing, black-or-white, and there's no room for screw-ups or mistakes. Perfectionism makes it hard to ever feel "done" or to give yourself the credit you deserve for where you are today. But no body fat percentage, the perfect tan, or external validation will award you with worthiness. We get to choose the next chapter in our own story and to believe that everything we need already exists inside of us.

14

THE POWER OF CHOICE

"The only way to the other side is through."

BY: JOHANNE WALKER

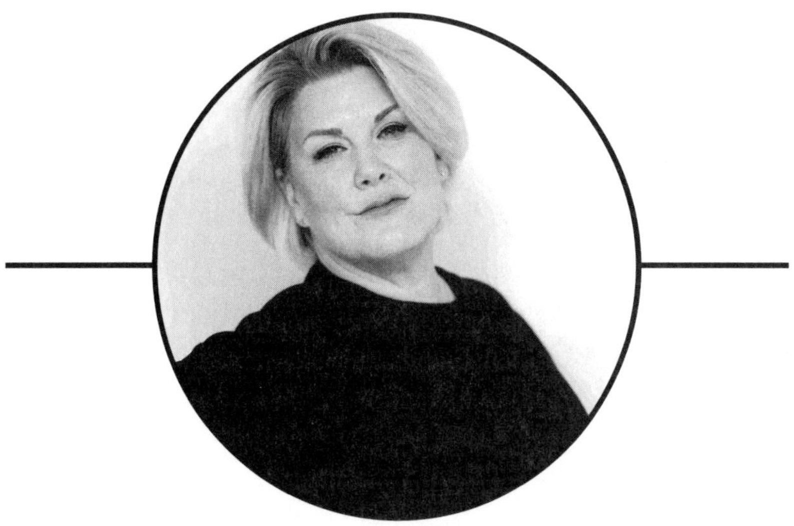

Johanne Walker is a woman with the most infectious energy who can get you believing in yourself before the conversation is over. Johanne channels her seeing-through-the-cracks superpower to help others meet themselves where they are. She's incredibly passionate about changing the conversation to cultivate a positive space and build a special connection with the self. She has created a movement to help all women look at themselves with an "I am enough" attitude.

Johanne's perspective includes connecting with community leaders and courageous women who are not afraid to embrace every part of themselves in order to help others in the community and the world. As the co-founder of the Women United Project, she focuses on creating a movement that will change the way we look at ourselves by creating a safe space for women to be vulnerable.

Johanne believes that when you're committed to change, life starts to look different. She encourages women to shift the way they approach things and realize that only they can make a difference in their own lives to change the way they think about themselves and their stories. She believes that the smallest of changes can lead to big results if we follow through with them and that if we could do it alone, we would've already done it

www.womenunitedproject.com

fb: women united project | ig: @womenunitedproject

When you say "yes" to something, you also say "no" to something else. When faced with one of life's challenges, in order to get to the other side, you need to go through! That means you have to do the work and love yourself fiercely, unapologetically, and consistently. It's the only way.

I love the rollercoaster of life. The thrill of the climb, the anticipation of what's next after you've reached the top, then the sudden dip where you're at the edge of your seat with your feet suspended in midair and your face pushed back, laughing and crying at the same time. And just when you think you've reached the end, it takes you right and then left in full throttle, slowing only to speed back up again, each turn joining your heart's rapid beating.

You think to yourself, "This is not so bad." You are facing your fears and embracing the ride; maybe you even start to enjoy yourself. You've just experienced the most heart-pumping, mind-blowing feeling, where every sensation in your body tells you that you're alive. Right when the ride ends, you catch yourself thinking, "I want to do it again. This time I'll keep my eyes open."

Welcome aboard the Walker Express.

I love the thrill of being alive, in love, and connected with myself and everyone around me. I have a modern-day family filled with laughs and joy — most of the time. I'm a mother to three adult children, a friend to an incredible stepdaughter, a grandmother to three of my grandchildren, and Jo to my two other grandkids. I am a serial entrepreneur with all things food, and I'm also a co-founder of an incredible community called the Women United Project, an online platform for women to embrace everything that we are and everything that we're not.

I've been my own witness and lived greatly to write this chapter. I raised three children through the teenage years and became friends with all of them (winning). I bridged two families with love and dedication. I survived divorce and found great love. I rocked the hell out of menopause with my sense of humor. I also love my body for all that I am and all that I am not, and I love sweating and moving my body, although that's been easier some years than others.

Taking care of myself starts with how I think and how I speak to myself, and I work at it every day. My inner dialogue affects everything in my life — if I'm not being nice to myself, how can I expect others to be nice to me? This is my daily practice. Although it's not an easy path, I work lovingly with myself. The biggest gift I've ever given myself is the gift of self-love.

In the immortal words of James Brown, *"I feel good / I knew that I would now / So good, so good, I got you."* These lyrics represent how I think about fueling my body; I love eating good food and feeling good about what I'm cooking and eating. Everything about food is exciting to me, from the way it looks to how it smells. It's just so fun to be creative in the kitchen! I know you may not believe me, but you can have great-tasting, good-for-you food — the best of both worlds.

I also love moving to feel the way I want to feel. You get to do what feels good for you, and it doesn't have to look the same for anyone else. From walking outside to dancing in your kitchen, exercises in your pool, yoga, strength training, and at-home workouts — you have choice! With all of these options, there's absolutely no reason not to move your body. That being said, I would be lying if I told you I never had excuses — and I have had a lot of good ones over the years. There's no easy way to convince yourself you need to move when you're feeling tired, run down, or straight-up exhausted. At that point, you have two options: feel fantastic or continue to feel like sh*t. The choice is yours. You are the boss of yourself, so ask yourself, "How do I want to feel? Now what?"

I am always listening to and taking care of my mind, body, and soul. I know a lot of people have said this before but it's incredibly true and relevant. There's no distinct separation between the three: the self is all connected. *Cool, right?* From my experience, how I move affects my mood, how I eat affects the clarify of my thoughts, and how I think affects every aspect of my body. This rings true not just in how I treat myself but also in how I show up for my children and my friends and in how I keep the love alive with my partner, Dan. People only take you as seriously as you take yourself.

Many of us get wrapped up in learning how to create a financial stability while exploring personal interests and curiosities. We invest time in seeking a life partner. We spend energy thinking about all the things we *should* be doing that we're not doing because we're trapped somewhere else, whether physically or mentally. It's time to say goodbye to this toxic energy: it's never been serving you. Instead, spend time with people who lift you up, who encourage you to do the things you always dreamed of, and who positively influence your choices. The time is now to rip the Band-aid off and tell yourself the truth. Get real and ask yourself, "What do I want?"

Trust me when I say that once you master your mind, you will love yourself like nobody else and make choices that lead you in the direction you want to go.

GET MOVING, MAMA

Let's back it up a bit and talk about moving our bodies when we're too tired, too busy, too *blah*. I know I've used every excuse in the book! I had three kids by the time I was twenty-five. I was sleep-deprived and had no break between feeding and changing diapers. To find a sliver of "me time," I had to go into the bathroom and close the door just for five minutes to be myself. All the while, we were living off one income with a full house and a marriage that wasn't fitting well anymore. I was a time bomb.

Yes, I know how my life got to that point — it was just always so much fun making these precious little gifts from heaven. I called these years the Character Development stage.

When I found yoga, it was out of pure desperation. This mama needed to chill out or someone was going to die. So I made my choice to get moving; I was determined to feel fantastic, no matter how exhausted I felt at that point. And slowly but surely, the dust in the air started to settle, or maybe I was just in a different headspace; I was gaining clarity and actually starting to enjoy the hustle-whirlwind life we had created.

Yoga saved my life and I was thrilled. Truth.

SHAKE WHAT YOUR MONEY GIVES YOU

Did I mention we were living on one income? Let me just tell you, it was difficult with so many mouths to feed and bodies to dress.

I wanted to provide a good life for my family, so I asked around for work. It needed to be the right fit. Eventually, I landed a cool gig in craft service (catering for the movie industry). My life has never been the same. In that job, I met the woman who changed my life — Susie Bradford. She was the founder of the company and not long after I started, we became the best of friends through our shared passion for business and yoga.

Life became steady. I was making money with hours that worked for my family. Everything changed so quickly for the better. I worked hard and kept my career moving in the right direction. I had gone from looking for part-time work to finding a career and a friendship that resonated with my soul. I started making great money, allowing for great perks like the ability to afford in-home care for my kids (the woman I hired was an absolute saint — she even did the laundry), travel, and purchase new homes and cars. I felt like I had won the lottery! This was so cool, right? I was busy and excelling - this unfortunately was a lot of change for my marriage to handle, but I was excited with the other aspects of my life.

Susie and I practiced yoga together every day for many, many years. Some days were easier than others. On the difficult days, we sat down to have coffee together and chat about our lives. We talked mostly of our steadfast approach to our yoga practice: how it was working so well and how I was feeling happy in my life and career, stronger and lighter by doing my daily practice. The direct effect of my daily practice became evident in all areas; my whole life shifted by doing just that one thing.

This practice of loving myself through yoga was hard, and not always convenient, but the payoff was way beyond anything I had expected. Each time I said yes to practice, I said no to a lot of things. No to staying up late and drinking too much alcohol. No to eating foods that made me feel heavy. And no to being treated like I didn't matter.

There were so many lessons I was learning about myself, lessons with hope, joy, and inner peace. And I liked what I saw. So I kept saying yes to me and my practice. Yoga allowed me freedom.

IT'S ALL ABOUT TIMING

Divorce, closing one business to start another (with Susie), closing that second business, moving, teenagers, heartbreak: at one point, I was full of sadness. My whole life had been turned upside down, everyone was mad at me, and I was mad at myself. It was like all the years of moving my body and feeling great had never happened. I was in turmoil and my entire family was suffering; we were all a mess. I couldn't bring myself to practice yoga, so I started running.

Running worked for me when I was angry and sad. It was challenging, and I didn't have to talk to anyone. I isolated myself and worked on perfecting my breathing technique. The best part was that there was no one to judge me. So believe me when I tell you, I ran a lot. It wasn't yoga, but I knew in my heart that it was what I needed at the time. My yoga mat has always been a reflection of what's going on in my life, and at the time, I was not interested in looking. Running gave me an outlet to express and release my pent-up emotions. Running allowed me freedom.

GETTING BACK ON TRACK

I was head over heels in love, the kids were growing up, and I was running, strength training, and practicing yoga daily. It had taken me a hot minute to sort my mess, but it's inevitable for real life and real conversations to get messy. My rebirth, for lack of a better word, was met with James Brown's *"I Feel Good"* once again. The first time I unrolled my yoga mat again was with Susie. Yoga was something she and I did together. We were a team.

Unfortunately, Susie was battling cancer — fighting for her life. I felt alone, sad, and angry that I couldn't do anything to help her. I cried the first time I stepped on my mat without Susie; I kid you not,

I was a falling-apart level of broken. All I could think about was my best friend and how dark the world would be without her light. With the mat as my mirror, I persisted. It went on for weeks: I'd unroll my mat, step on it, cry, and think about Susie. Then, one day, I stopped crying. I believed that I could heal her from my mat with the love I had for her. So I started practicing and dedicating my yoga to her. I later enrolled in teacher training. I was committed to my practice and to making Susie feel loved and supported. We were still on this journey together; it was just different than what we had in mind.

Susie lost her battle with cancer and I miss her every day. I still dedicate my practice to her — feeling grateful to have known her, to be healthy and mobile, to be able to move my body the way I want, and to have a great life with my family.

On the rollercoaster ride of my life, I have gone in and out of that James Brown song in my head. It's not easy choosing me every day but it's so necessary. I knew for sure that if I didn't choose me, nobody else would do it for me. My life has carried me through a full spectrum of emotions and I wouldn't have it any other way.

On this crazy, up-and-down ride of a lifetime, the only way to the end is through. And whether you keep your eyes open, peek through the cracks of your fingers, or shut them completely shut — the choice is yours.

I repeat: *the choice is yours.*

IT'S YOU — IT'S ALWAYS BEEN YOU

Choose nice words when you speak to yourself; choose to move your body; choose to look at yourself in the mirror (or on your mat like me) with gentleness; choose feeling good over feeling bad; choose to express how you feel; and always choose love.

These choices are a practice, just like yoga; it comes more easily some days than others, just like a rollercoaster ride can leave you feeling differently than the ride before. Make the choices that make you feel good because taking care of yourself creates room for everything else to work. Get your calendar out and schedule in time for *you*.

With a consistent practice of self-love and care, you will feel better every day. Without such a practice, you will just fall to the wayside. If you struggle with establishing a self-love and care practice, join a studio, ask a girlfriend for help, and connect to other women. We're stronger together.

How you choose to wield your power speaks volumes about the kind of person that you are — including yourself from the past, yourself in the future, and yourself at this very moment.

I've always said that when you choose yourself first, when you put yourself first, you consistently rise above because you hold yourself accountable to do what you were meant to do. You're also raising the bar for how you look at yourself and how others look at you. You're walking into your own power, so step up to the plate, take your shot, and fulfill your destiny.

I want to leave you with this nugget: by embracing every part of myself (even the parts I thought I couldn't), I was able to love myself back to happiness — to home — where my family belongs.

Through yoga, I've finally met myself where I am. And I am home.

15

HOME IS WHERE YOUR BODY IS

"Moving your body daily is the catalyst to your freedom."

BY: JOCELYN HINZ

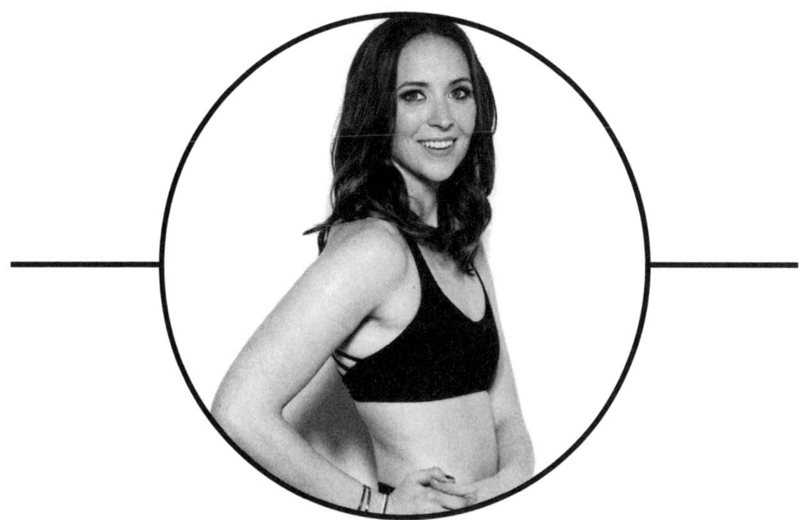

Jocelyn Hinz is obsessed with holding space for you to explore your real truths, strengths, body, and movement. As a successful entrepreneur who quit the corporate crawl, Jocelyn is known for creating dynamic yoga classes focused on the real feel, cultivating conversations about living wildly in alignment with your heart, and advocating for less stigma in coming back home to your body.

Jocelyn works with young women who want to cultivate a deeper connection to their body, mind, and spirit without sacrificing their identity. Through the use of doTERRA essential oils, movement, and the cultivation of intuition and trust, she is helping women wake up to their own potential.

Jocelyn is the founder of a global essential oil collective. She thrives on dark chocolate and red wine and wishes that every sunset would get a parade. Jocelyn aims to bring the balance back between flow and hustle, green juice and wine, take-out and organic groceries — that balance is where her life lives.

www.jocelynhinz.com

ig: @joce.hinz

My journey home to my body has been riddled with experiences that have added texture to my life. I continue to be schooled in how to create a deeper relationship with my cells, and my intention here is to create a space for you to explore your body, too. I want these words to spark a revolution inside of you and to drum up the brilliance that is feeling quiet in this moment.

I am fully and wholeheartedly walking alongside you, connecting to this liberation of my cells. I have spent over half of my life learning to cultivate a loving relationship with my body. For the longest time, I didn't know how to establish such a relationship because I couldn't connect to a powerful example of it within my life. Society tells us from an early age that we need to fix what is wrong with us. The outside world, media, Hollywood, and Photoshop do a great job showing us how to both stand out and fit in in terms of what we should wear, how we should act, what we should eat, how long our hair should be, how skinny our jeans should be, how skinny we should be. These outside voices are experts in creating a fake image that we are not-so-subtly told to strive for. What the media and societal norms do not teach us is how to cultivate trust in ourselves and our voice.

How do we become the curator of the relationship with our body?

When I was fifteen, I would do sit-ups in my basement after meals because I wanted to see my abs. I would pay attention to what the other girls at school were eating and how they were dressing. I was born with an athletic body shape and a metabolism that is always firing because ever since I could walk, I was running. I played on an incredible number of sports teams throughout my childhood and into my late twenties, including soccer, baseball, volleyball, badminton, and cross-country running. Then I explored basketball at the club level and the college level. My body has always supported me physically, but just because I was strong and slim doesn't mean I had a healthy relationship with myself. Just because I fit into my jeans doesn't mean I looked in the mirror and loved what I saw.

Let me be clear: I treated my body like an absolute wreck as I navigated high school, college, and life post-studies. As I was testing boundaries as a teenager, I started to drink and party like it was the only thing on my calendar. I became a pro at going to school and training during the week and then losing my mind in a shot glass on the weekends. That was how I lived my life for almost ten years. That means, a decade of my life was devoted to being numb, cellular terror, squashed intuition and a routine that didn't give me any space to breathe.

I didn't understand what being healthy meant. I thought I was healthy because I could challenge myself athletically. I thought I was healthy because I got good grades and achieved high academic status. I thought I was healthy because I had a stable family. I thought I was healthy because I ate whole wheat bread. I thought I was healthy because my jeans fit. What I didn't recognize at the time was that health means different things for every single person in every single season of our lives. Being healthy takes on different shapes and is such a beautiful, individualized experience that we get to explore within ourselves. Our health is in constant flux, and what makes us feel good one moment may not the next. This point of flux is where we get to flex our trust muscle and roll out our own welcome mat to come back into our body by asking the right questions of ourselves.

I stayed in constant movement because I didn't know who I was or where I belonged in the world. I moved my body to escape, not to curate. My relationship with movement started to feel heavy. I quit playing my team sports and went to the gym again. I became that girl in the gym just filling up her water bottle, stretching in the mirror, and walking on the treadmill. I didn't have the capacity to push myself any longer, and I didn't want to.

I felt ultra-aware of how disconnected I had become from myself and how numb the world felt. I decided to try yoga — again. I should preface this by saying that I did go to a hot yoga class with my athletic therapist in college once. I wore a cotton t-shirt and basketball shorts and had to rent a mat and towel. I remember filling up my water bottle from their filtered water station thinking that this place was Zen as shit and I absolutely didn't belong there. I legitimately walked out with half of my bodily fluids left on the mat. So technically, when I walked into my local Modo studio, it was my second shot at hot yoga. All I knew was that I needed to create a space in my life where I could feel and connect to something bigger than myself again.

The feeling that pulsed through my veins when I left class was liberation. I was and continue to be the sweatiest person on the mat, but I felt something. I felt an electrical jolt run through my body that I hadn't experienced before. It was like my nervous system was carried back into alignment, and my body energetically picked up that feeling and needed more. I went back the next day and the following thirty days after that. I was so drawn to this practice of coming back into my body on my mat. It was the only place where I could shut out the world and just connect to my breath. This felt foreign to me but also synergistically aligned. My body ate it up. The practice was challenging and gentle, and I learned how to breathe as I turned the dial up on my awareness. I unlocked the next chapter of my life that month, and I felt it.

The physical practice landed so naturally in my body and after a few months of regular practice, the emotional softening followed. I was starting to be more mindful about what went into and onto my body. This is the side benefit of movement — you start to care, you start to feel and heal. It may happen unconsciously in the beginning, but your awareness grows with you and then it becomes deliberate.

It only took me about six months to recognize that I needed yoga in my life full time. I signed up for a yoga teacher training, quit my job, and drove to Montreal for a full thirty days. When I feel something deep in my bones, I don't mess around. Decisions are made, bags are packed, accommodations are booked, and the plan is in motion. My life was forever altered in this space. I left behind the version of the girl who was numb, broken, and defeated, and I woke up to this big, bold, beautiful, encompassing life.

I feel very aware of my own privilege when it comes to my story. Financially I was able to count on my parents for help. I was able to quit my job because I knew I could just get another; I knew I would land on my feet because the world is set up for me to do that easily. I understand and connect with the fact that not everyone experiences this birthright, that the world and how we are able to show up and experience it is drastically different for people who don't share my skin colour. I want my words to reflect the experience of being open to coming home and committing to show up for your soul in whatever space you are currently in.

Moving on my mat became my daily ritual. It was my new drug of choice, and I couldn't get enough. I started to feel into my body again, to celebrate its strength, to flex this new sensitivity for who I was becoming. With this new movement came deep healing. Our individual experiences, our generational past, our lineage, and all of the hardships that come with those things — all of this lands in our body, in our tissues, our bones, our muscles, our structure. It lands there energetically and when we become aware of it, we only have one way through. Lean in and get dirty with it.

I started to turn over and scrub through not only the ten-plus years of neglecting my body and mind but also deep generational wounds. It felt intense but the more I explored this in my life, the deeper the healing became. I would never suggest to you that we all process life and heal in the same way because that is not the truth. What I do want to suggest are three keys that helped me open the doors to my own truest self; I want to leave you these keys to let yourself back into your own home.

PAUSE

There is a gift in pausing, taking a deep breath and feeling the air move through your nose and expand into your lungs. There is a gift in feeling your feet on the ground and the warmth of the sun on your face. There is a gift in asking for what you need in this exact moment. There is a gift in tapping out of your thinking mind and into your feeling heart.

Pausing creates a waterfall effect in our body in which we get to check in and evaluate. We create names for feelings based on the vibration they hold in our body so we can address those feelings as they rise, look at them, hold them up to the light, and understand them. We need to cry in the bath with them or sweat them out of our cells; we need to use our tools like powerful plant essential oils, movement, and journaling practices to create heat with our feelings so that one day, we can see it all differently. We can envelop those feelings with love and understanding, holding them in our body without being triggered and arriving at a place of wholeness once again. We never fully let any of our experiences go, but what we can do is cradle them in our arms and whisper sweet words to them so they no longer hold power over us.

I didn't know it at the time but when I walked into that yoga studio and committed to my practice, I unconsciously created space for myself to pause, to feel, to heal, and to transform. I needed to feel my body sweat, to experience life-altering cellular shifts, to be led into a place of gentleness, to heighten my awareness, and to forgive myself.

My mantra became *move, feel, heal, and then teach.*

BOUNDARIES

There are so many versions of ourselves scattered through our own story. Someone once told me that I wasn't at all who they remembered, and I was all like, *"Hell yes, sister!"* If we are to truly experience this life and all its offerings, then of course we need to stretch and grow and move and surrender to this process of evolving. Of course we will change emotionally and physically and spiritually. Of course we will shed old stories of who we think we are and should be.

Some days I felt like I was changing and healing and moving so quickly that I didn't know who I was. Other days I felt like I was moving backward and that time was standing still. I had to keep reminding myself that I didn't get to this space of disconnect, hurt, and pain overnight, so how could I expect to shift to the next chapter so fast? I had to sit with it, feel it, process, and move forward. I had to create boundaries around my time and my space. After all, I wasn't sitting in a robe on a mountaintop, healing and drinking tea. I was living my regular day to day, doing the things needed to keep a home and relationship and new puppy alive.

Being vigilant about who and what we allow into this new space we are creating is the epitome of creating boundaries. You are allowed to take time for yourself, you are allowed to slow down, you are allowed to flow with the seasons, and you are allowed to move with your cycle. You are allowed to say who gets a free pass into your space. Creating boundaries is imperative to healing.

SWEAT

This life is too sacred to not participate in fully, and moving your body daily is the catalyst to your freedom.

One more time for the sister in the back: moving your body daily is the catalyst to your freedom.

There is a season to rest, there is a season to prepare, and there is a season to move. Humans are not wired to be in flow three hundred and sixty-five days a year. It is just not possible; that is when we get burnt out or injured. What we can always commit to, however, is being our own best friend, having our own back, listening to the subtleties of our energy, and making our move from there. Would you tell your best friend that she sucks and is the worst? No. Be kind to yourself, all right? Give yourself some grace for rest. Release the shame; there is no space for that vibration in your body.

If right now you are in a season in which your self-talk is heavy or your vibration feels funky, take your body out on a date and move it around in whatever way feels right. This might be a yoga class, a barre class, or a run; maybe you throw some weights around, maybe you dance until you are beat or go for a long walk. You, girlfriend, have your own back and you know exactly what season you are in. Move accordingly.

There is space in your breath to be kind to yourself today and to trust that the freedom you are seeking is already living inside of you. *You* are remarkable, *your* body is bangin', *your* mind is intelligent, you are an incredible woman and friend and sister and aunt and (fur) mom, and *you* can create a new level of freedom in your life. When you embrace your truth and uniqueness and authenticity and all that you are, your freedom looks like radiance and you belong to yourself again. You are finally home.

16

THE CHOICE IS ALWAYS YOURS

"When action mirrors words, the unbelievable appears."

BY: PAULINE CABALLERO

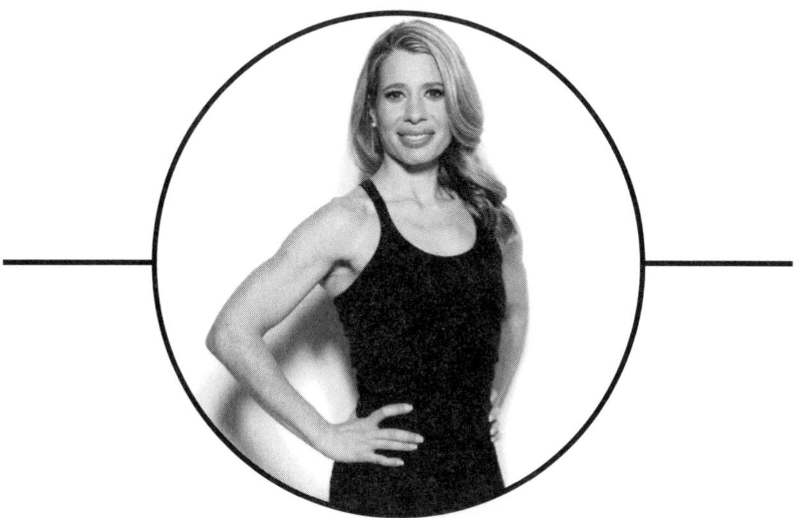

Led by her interest in developing others, Pauline Caballero is always looking for ways to create opportunities for people to thrive and live their best lives. She is a wife and a mom of two boys, as well as the co-founder of Power Yoga Canada, a hot vinyasa studio brand. She has also held various corporate executive positions. Pauline is interested in eradicating the belief that we must all find balance and would rather help people accept the organized chaos that we call life. You can find Pauline practicing yoga with her youngest son or watching her eldest son play hockey. She is a rink rat with a passion and love for sport and fitness.

www.poweryogacanada.com

ig: @paulinecaballero

Life is just too busy. I hope one day I will find time to work out. Those disempowering statements ran over and over in my head like a bad Netflix show. I had years of excuses and reasons (and good ones, I might add) for why it was not the right time to work on myself. It was as if I were just waiting patiently for my fitness fairy godmother to come whisk me off my feet and lead me to a land where I worked out religiously and was in perfect form. Well, let me cut to the end of that story: there was not enough hope in the world that would turn my thinking into results. Simply put, if I wanted a different result in life, I would have to work for it.

As a former competitive figure skater and the owner of multiple yoga studios, exercise has always been a part of my life, although this was truer for some years than for others. What I have discovered throughout the years is that although I love to exercise, I also *need* to exercise. It is the thing that regulates my life, the one thing I can count on to maintain my mental health. Exercise is my lifeline and whether it is scientifically proven or completely a placebo effect, what I have come to know to be true is that moving and sweating *every single day* has saved my life.

Perhaps because exercise was always present in my life, though, I never thought I had to schedule it in or make it a priority. Well, like all things, if you don't put your attention on them, even good habits fade away. Despite being the owner of a yoga studio, I could not create a consistent movement practice. I am also a horrible cook and an executive turned yoga teacher turned executive again, and I found it challenging to establish a regular exercise and health routine.

Five years ago, I found myself neck-deep with a one-year-old and a seven-year-old. I was sick all the time. It was a vicious cycle of taking as much cold medicine as possible, masking the illness, getting through work, flying home, and then being out of commission for days. I did this over and over and over again. No matter what season it was, I was guaranteed to be sick. Looking back, I cannot believe that I allowed myself to operate that way. My body was tired, and I hoped that one day I would feel better, one day I would have the energy to stay awake while I played with my sons. I was suffering from chronic fatigue but I simply kept hoping that my poor health would turn around, chalking it up to a barrage of excuses. *I am working too hard. Traveling is tiring.* I can't tell you how many times I told myself, "I just have to get through this one thing," but that quickly turned into "I just have to get through this day, this week, this year." My life was running me. I was not making choices; I just was the victim of my life. Until one day, it all changed.

After my kids started school in September 2015, I decided that I needed a new way of operating. I was spending my life focused on other people's agendas and not my own. I ensured that everyone had their needs met but I was not affording myself the same level of commitment. Bottom line: I was not honoring my word to myself. I wanted to make fitness a priority; I mean, I owned yoga studios and worked in the well-being industry, so why would I not make my own health a priority? The problem was that I was unwilling to concede that I had failed at juggling it all.

When I opened the first Power Yoga Canada studio in 2009 with my business partner, Kinndli McCollum, I was taking a stand in how I wanted to operate in my life. I was throwing caution to the wind and deciding that things, job titles, and "stuff" would not define me. My previous life as an executive had made me feel completely run down from trying to prove myself and trying to make it. At the time, I would have blamed my mother, saying that she constantly pushed me to prove myself and compared me to others and that this had made me tired of the rat race. I know better today and am clear my burnout has nothing to do with how my mom raised me. She was simply doing the best job she knew how to do and was hoping to push me to be the best version of myself.

Opening that first yoga studio back in 2009 represented my commitment to health and well-being. The problem was that it did not last. Here I was just over five years later, back where I started — on my knees. I was drowning for a new way to function and be in the world, but I was also suffering from chronic fatigue and lacked the willingness to believe that there was another way. Worst of all, I felt like a complete fraud. I owned studios and here I was, not committed to practicing, happy to promote healthy living as long as I didn't have to follow the routine myself. It is here on my knees that all the healing began and I made the commitment to creating a new, sustainable path for myself.

The yo-yo years were so extreme and happened so frequently that it was as if I expected them and used them to shame myself. *Oh, here you are again, Pauline; see, you couldn't keep your weight down or your mental state intact.* I kept failing because it was a way for me to sabotage and punish myself. I allowed myself to believe that I didn't deserve anything good or whole or complete. It wasn't until I accepted myself for who I was and for who I wasn't, for my flaws and for my strengths, for my body and for my thoughts, that I was actually able to live into a new way of being and operating.

The very first thing I did was get back onto my mat. Every day. This was a coming home for me and more importantly, it created stability for my mental well-being. I recruited my husband to be my biggest supporter. Then I followed four simple steps (shared in the next section). At the time I wasn't consciously completing these steps; I was simply in action. I was so committed to creating new habits that I just began. I took the calendar and counted out exactly one hundred days, and then I wrote out how I would sweat each day.

My journey back to fitness was a long road, but I was more committed to my goal than I was to my excuses, so no matter where I was, I sweated. Hotel rooms, at home after putting the kids down — I no longer allowed there to be any reason to *not* honor my word to myself.

Here are the four steps I took to shift from a life of survival to a life of thriving by focusing on and prioritizing health through fitness.

STEP ONE: TELL THE TRUTH!

I had to understand what I was most disappointed in and come totally clean about it. To tell the truth to myself about aspects of my life in which I was completely inauthentic. To be honest about when I was saying I wanted to do something but then simply not doing it. That list hurt. I wanted to be disciplined and go to the gym every day, but the truth was, I slept through my alarm.

Where are you saying you want something but being unwilling to take the actions to achieve it? Journal on that!

STEP TWO: WHO DO I WANT TO BE ONE HUNDRED DAYS FROM NOW?

In order for me to live into a better future, I needed to create it. Do this brief exercise for yourself. First right down today's date. Now count out one hundred days from today. Write that day (month, day, and year) down. Close your eyes and simply breathe. I want you to imagine what you are doing on that one hundredth day. What are you wearing? Who are you with? What are you saying? What are you not saying? Who are you being? Once you get a sense of who that person is, open your eyes and write it down. Be detailed and vividly describe everything you saw, felt, and heard. Your opening sentence can look something like this: On [insert date] I am . . .

STEP THREE: MAKE A PLAN.

Once I looked at who I wanted to be in one hundred days, it was quite evident that there was a huge gap between that person and who I currently was. My goal was to work out every day; however, nothing on my calendar supported that initiative. How was I to achieve my goal if I didn't have a clear plan to execute it? I quickly took action.

I first had some problems to overcome. For example, I am a mom, and the kids' activities happen in the evenings. It was not practical or realistic to think I could schedule a workout in the evenings. Problem number two was that I have a job. That means I could not attend a 9:30am yoga class either. So I went off to find a class that happened before everyone woke up in my household. That proved to not be easy, until one day it was. One thing that I have learned on this journey to freedom with my fitness regime is that I must be more committed to my goals than to my excuses or obstacles. There are a million reasons why I can't do something. I had to develop the strength to stay committed to what I wanted to accomplish; only then would all the pieces begin to fall into place. I found a local gym that offered a 5:15am weekday class, and I negotiated a time that my husband would be comfortable with me working out on Saturdays and Sundays. Most importantly, I marked these times in my calendar and asked my family for support. I recruited the people in my life into the game I was playing, which was working out every single day for one hundred days.

Now it is time for you to take the time to determine the following:

1. What needs to be in your calendar? What time needs to be carved out?
2. What agreements do you need to update? For example, do you need to communicate your plans to your significant other? To your family? To your co-workers? To your boss?
3. Who do you need to support you with this plan? Have you asked them for their support?

Once you have answered these questions and are confident with your plan, you are ready for the final step.

STEP FOUR: WORK THE PLAN.

This statement sounds easier than it is, but for me, it was the most rewarding accomplishment. In one hundred days, I finally did what I said I was going to do for myself, and I have not looked back. I faced so many obstacles, challenges, and roadblocks along the way, and things didn't always go to plan. However, it was my time to get creative. A missed workout turned into a thirty-minute video workout in my pajamas with my boys because they were committed to seeing me win my game. I found that when you recruit others to join your game, they become your support system. My family became my reason to stick to my word. I invite you to work the plan by taking what you have written seriously. Ask yourself, "If I worked this plan, what would be possible for me?" There is a miracle waiting for you on the other side of one hundred days. The question is, are you up for it?

Today, I have found the freedom to move every day in order to maintain my quality of life. The habit of daily workouts has stuck for me. Some days are longer than others, but the practice of no days off, or as I like to say, "all days on," has stuck. The results I have experienced are profound. I find myself sleeping through the entire night. I am conscious about what I put into my mouth and how I fuel my body, without having to put myself on a strict diet. Most importantly, my mental health is stable. I come from a family in which depression and schizophrenia are common, and I've found exercise to be the best prescription ever to deal with these risks. In fact, I have deemed it my life-long prescription. My daily fitness ritual has become the structure I needed to give me the freedom to be creative and boundless in other areas of my life. Structuring my mornings has given me the liberty to work through my lunch and play at night with my kids. I have found that by making myself a priority and sticking with my plan, I have freed up my entire family.

On that day in 2015, I realized that no one was coming to save me; I would have to save myself. The commitment required of me is best described by Johann Wolfgang Von Goethe:

> Until one is committed, there is hesitancy, the chance to draw back, always ineffectiveness. Concerning all acts of initiative and creation, there is one elementary truth the ignorance of which kills countless ideas and splendid plans: that the moment one definitely commits oneself, then providence moves too. All sorts of things occur to help one that would never otherwise have occurred. A whole stream of events issues from the decision, raising in one's favor all manner of unforeseen incidents, meetings and material assistance which no man could have dreamed would have come his way. Whatever you can do or dream you can, begin it. Boldness has genius, power and magic in it. Begin it now.

Where do you need to level up your commitments? What do you need to stop doing? What do you need to start doing? Are you exhausted of hearing your own excuses? It is only when you make the choice to shift your language and your being that you can change.

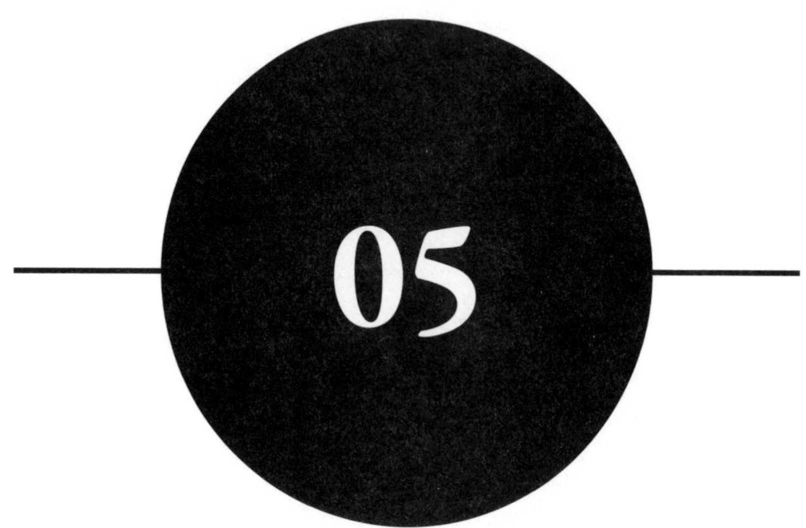

THE FREEDOM TO HELP OTHERS

17

HOW FITNESS SHAPED ME INTO THE PERSON I AM TODAY

"Size doesn't matter, but mindset does."

BY: KAREN SWYSZCZ

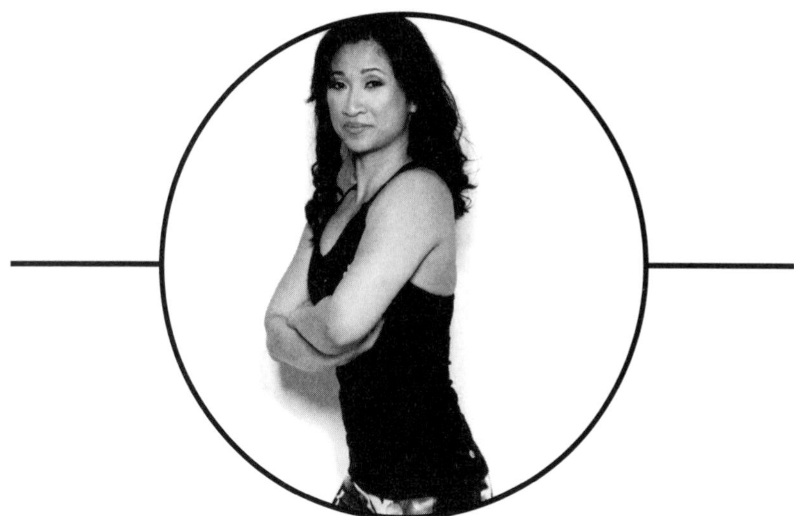

As much as Karen Swyszcz loved running around and chasing other kids on the playground, being active was not encouraged in her family. Her gym rat life began during university where she would do only cardio-related activities: running, spinning, and swimming at the local YMCA.

Karen was then introduced to Bodypump, a barbell workout class, and instantly fell in love. She loved it so much that she went through the training to become an instructor. As an introvert, being an instructor enables Karen to come out of her shell and take on an entirely different persona.

Karen also has a love for writing. Her blog, Makinthebacon, started in 2012 as a passion project to escape the monotony of her government job. Little did she know that this blog would significantly transform her life. It enabled her to make a bold career change and not too long after to start her own consulting business in blogging and social media.

Karen has the natural ability to seek and create opportunities. She is passionate about helping others tell their story and believes your passions can help you make the bacon.

https://makinthebacon.com

fb, ig, t: @makinthebacon1

Sports did not have a place in our household. My parents' wish for me was to spend my time chasing good grades rather than chasing any kind of football, soccer ball, or volleyball. After all, good grades meant a good college, which meant a good job, which meant a better life — and that was the reason they both came to Canada [separately] from the Philippines in the first place, to create better opportunities for themselves.

Although I, their active eldest daughter, was constantly running around at birthday parties and hanging out on the playground monkey bars, they steered my focus and attention toward keeping my nose in the books. Perhaps they were overprotective. Perhaps they viewed sports as "just for boys," as many people did back then.

I ignored their worries and concerns and still participated in a few team sports in high school: cross-country running one year, rugby another. It wasn't until university that I dipped my toe into the fitness world by exploring the local community swimming pool and later, as I grew bolder, spinning and running. I wasn't proficient at any of these activities by any means, but I had taken my first shaky steps toward a fitness journey that would transform my body, my business, and my life.

I just didn't know it yet.

HOW THE FITNESS ADDICTION STARTED

I'll never forget the first time I took a BodyPump class. A good friend from university, Andrea, introduced me to the class. For those of you who may not know, BodyPump is a group barbell workout that involves a lot of repetitions with light to moderate weights. Like most women, I was mildly (read: super) terrified of becoming "bulky" if I so much as looked at a pair of weights, so I used the lightest option available. Even that felt impossible.

I can't remember what specifically made me want to keep coming back, but I believe it was the combination of great instructors, music, and working together as a group toward a common goal. As soon as I got a full-time job after graduation, I joined the gym so I could attend the group fitness classes after work and get that hit of adrenaline I never knew I was missing.

After attending BodyPump as a participant for almost a year, I thought about becoming an instructor. I love learning, trying new things, and taking on new challenges, so I felt that getting my instructor certification made sense as the next challenge. I went for the required two-day training and basically had my ass handed to me. I was fit, but I needed to get "instructor fit"— an entirely different level of being in shape that felt superhuman and therefore impossible. Fortunately, what I lacked in muscles I made up for with determination, and I was resolved to improve.

After the initial training, I spent a lot of time team teaching with more experienced instructors to get used to teaching in front of members and being up on stage. In order to become certified, you have to film a video of yourself teaching an entire class. Trying to talk while lifting heavy weights is no walk in the park. Add in having to motivate and coach people, make sure everyone is moving safely, cue the next movement, and demonstrate proper technique, while having *all* of that happen in time with the music, and you have an instant recipe for a very stressed and overwhelmed Karen.

As someone who is an introvert and painfully shy, I struggled to be outgoing and energetic on stage. I failed the video submission part the first time around, which devastated me. I had spent so much time and energy learning the choreography and filming multiple times. My pride was as sore as my body and I wanted to give up. I dreaded the thought of having to go through the constant practicing and filming all over again. However, there was this little voice in my head that said, "Don't give up. Try again. Come on, Karen." I decided to persevere and ended up passing the second time around.

HOW BEING A GROUP FITNESS INSTRUCTOR TRANSFORMED ME

I knew becoming a group fitness instructor would take my personal fitness to a whole new level, but I never expected the mental transformation that accompanied the title. Confidence and courage were qualities that were completely unknown to me but with which I now became acquainted. I now realize how much courage it took for that sheltered, first-generation Canadian girl to do what she did.

Pushing my physical limitations, getting up in front of a class, and leading those people toward their own transformations was brave, to say the least. In addition to providing a significant personal transformation, teaching these classes has helped me get through some difficult times in my life (the loss of a loved one, my less-than-ideal job situation, and my lack-of-money situation). Whatever issues or problems I had, I knew I had to check them at the door because dwelling on them would be detrimental to my teaching. The classes taught me how to shift my priorities and my focus, and how to do it fast.

HOW I SHAPED MYSELF INTO A LEADER

It's crazy to think how much of an impact I've had on people's lives. My class might be the one time my members can shut out everything else or their chance to be social in a very welcoming environment. Each of my classes has its own little community, and I have witnessed many friendships form through group fitness. I have also witnessed the incredible transformation of some of the members. To see them go from their first class to lifting heavier weights or doing pushups on their toes brings me nothing but pride and joy.

I never really considered myself to be a leader; I've always seen myself more as a follower. In my classes, it may only be for an hour, but for that hour, I am leading people, many of whom have been coming to my classes for years. It is my responsibility (a responsibility I take very seriously) to challenge them each week and lead them through a safe, yet effective workout. Even after an amazing class, I'll sometimes stop and think, *Was there anything I could have done better?*

In addition to the physical energy, a lot of mental energy goes into teaching a fitness class, which is why I like to relax and have some alone time after I teach. Trying to learn brand new choreography while still teaching the older choreography for two different types of classes (BodyPump and BodyAttack) every quarter is always stressful.

More often than not, I ask myself how I will ever learn it all. As my members' fearless leader, I am down in the trenches with them, muscles burning, sweat dripping down my face. There is nothing more satisfying when we are working through the last few reps of a tough track together. They rely on me to help them get through the workout, and we keep each other accountable.

I feel I have a responsibility to not only talk the talk but also walk the walk. Some people think teaching the classes is a good enough workout, but it's not the same. At the end of the day, it's more the members' workout than my own. In addition to teaching, I try to get in my own workouts once or twice a week, whether it's doing my own thing or participating in a class that I don't teach.

I'll be honest, there are some days when I don't feel up to teaching, days when I would rather just do my own workout. However, I know the moment the music starts and I'm up on stage, I am good to go. I get such a high from leading people through a workout.

Members often say that I make it look so easy or that they can't believe someone my size (I'm petite) could be so strong, but that strength has been built up over many years of teaching. They also don't see the amount of time and effort I put into creating a workout I feel will challenge them every time. As an instructor, you end up wearing many hats. You are not just an instructor: you are a motivator. You are a performer. You are an athlete. You need to demonstrate strength, agility, endurance, power, and proper technique. Every. Single. Time.

HOW FITNESS HELPS MY BUSINESS

Although it is not technically recognized by the fitness community as a sport, I am an expert "juggler." It's a skill I developed when I became a solopreneur — I have a lot of balls up in the air all the time, and it's my responsibility to keep them all safely moving, just like I have a responsibility to keep my members safely moving during a workout.

For many people, a ball that often gets dropped is making time to exercise. As a fitness instructor, I'm able to fit exercise into my schedule on a regular basis. It is a non-negotiable for me. The gym is where I go when I need a break from the computer or need to get out of the house. After a workout, my mind becomes clearer and I am able to focus better.

My years as a fitness instructor have provided me with essential skills for not just starting but also sustaining my business. All those years of being on stage have given me the mental and emotional strength to speak in front of audiences and facilitate workshops for my business. I still get nervous, but I tell myself that people are here to learn from me and become motivated.

Having your own business can feel like a grueling workout that never ends. Entrepreneurs are constantly exhausted, mentally, physically, and emotionally. This is where personal workouts come in and provide the energy to withstand the long, challenging days. Sometimes when I'm in the middle of a tough set, I'll be thinking, *I can get through whatever business problem I'm having.*

I'm still human though. I would be lying if I said I don't find it difficult even now to balance a business, my fitness classes, and the courses I teach at the college, let alone having a life. There are days when I am mentally exhausted from working on my business and all I want to do is sit on the couch, eat fries, and binge watch Netflix. After all, fitness professionals are people, too.

HOW I EVOLVED AND HOW YOU CAN TRANSFORM, TOO

Trying a group fitness class, especially one that seems pretty intense, can be very intimidating. I'd like to offer one simple piece of advice — just try. We may be at different levels of fitness, but we are all there for the same reason. We all want to improve our health and well-being.

Group fitness is such a great confidence-builder, and that same confidence will slowly integrate into other important areas of your life, personally and professionally.

After becoming a group fitness instructor, I feel like I can take on anything and overcome any obstacle. Being up on stage and leading a workout has increased my confidence tremendously in the gym, outside of the studio, and life in in general. I used to be terrified of going to the area of the gym with the free weights or of using the weight machines. I eventually realized that I have every right to be there with the guys and I shouldn't feel intimidated. I should be proud of how far I've come in my fitness journey and of the fact that I am one tiny but tough female.

HOW WE ARE ALL A WORK(OUT) IN PROGRESS

Despite having been an instructor for many years and seeing a dramatic increase in my strength, endurance, and power, I sometimes feel like I am not fit or strong enough and that I could do better. I compare myself to other fitness instructors from time to time, and social media can only intensify the comparison game.

Sometimes I even think I need to be more outgoing and bubblier in general, but that's not who I am naturally. I have thought the same thing in my business, that I needed to be a certain way. The truth is, though, we all have different personalities and styles. The most important thing is that we all have a love for fitness.

I hear a lot excuses from people as to why they don't have the time to exercise — lack of money, lack of time, it's too hard, I have kids, it hurts, and on and on. More often than not, I feel like these excuses are such nonsense. We make time for what's important to us, and it's important to make ourselves a priority. Nobody is born fit. We all have to start somewhere and work at it. Yes, some of us have to work harder than others, but we all can work (and work out) anywhere and everywhere.

HOW FITNESS MAKES YOU STRONGER: NOT JUST PHYSICALLY, BUT MENTALLY

Working out is not just about looking good. It's about the positive feelings we get from exercise and tying those good feelings into everything we set out to achieve in life.

In business and in life, there will always be obstacles and setbacks. Being a group fitness instructor has given me the mental toughness to break through these challenges and move forward, continuing on my journey to success. Thanks to my fitness routine, I am not as afraid of taking risks or asking for what I want in my business.

If you had told the cardio-only version of me many years ago that in the future, I would be a fitness inspiration to others and run my own consulting business, I would have shaken my head and laughed in disbelief. And yet here I am, many years later, sharing my many stories of failures and successes, all thanks to fitness. Even though fitness is only one part of my life and not my actual business, it was the initial step to shaping me into the person I am today.

I encourage you to make fitness a part of your journey and look forward to the opportunities it will create, the paths it will take you on, and the destinations it will lead you to.

18

WHEN WE LEARN, WE TEACH

"Every great dream begins with a dreamer. Always remember you have within you the strength, the patience and the passion to reach for the stars, to change the world." - Harriet Tubman

BY: CAROL HANLEY

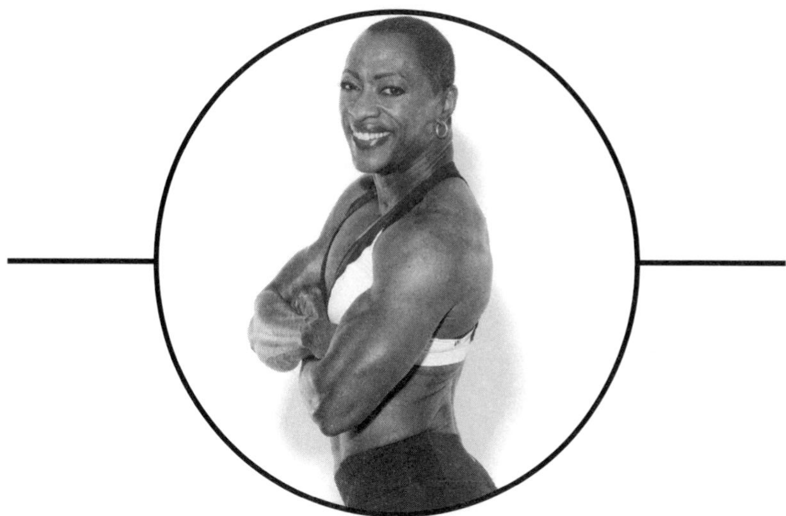

Armed with both determination and stubbornness, Carol Hanley set out to achieve her first place ranking in the Canadian Women's Middleweight competitive bodybuilding forum. After competing for three years, she not only achieved a first place ranking in Canada but also went on to take first place in North America in two different Middleweight classes. What a journey it has been for this Canadian "Iron Princess," who proudly embraces both her hometown of Basseterre St. Kitts, and Mississauga, Ontario.

Carol grew up in a disciplined environment with a grandfather who was chief of police and a devoted grandmother. She attended a private grade school in St. Kitts before finishing her studies in Montreal, Quebec. After first pursuing post-secondary studies in the areas of medicine, she found herself drawn to technology and finished her degree in computer science. She is currently an executive managing director of software development.

Carol's love and interest in bodybuilding started at a very young age with reading magazines and producing sketches of muscle-bound comic book heroes. She continued to follow the sport as a fan and dreamed from the sidelines until finally following her passion and stepping on stage. Carol was no stranger to sports, as she was an avid athlete: track and field, volleyball, basketball, and tennis. Carol's decision to embark on this competitive pathway came about after talking to a fellow competitor who took the time to encourage her to pursue her dreams. After continuously winning in various classes for five years, she took home the coveted IFBB Pro Card and become a Professional Athlete.

www.hanco-tech.com

ig: @ironprincess007

"Each time a woman stands up for herself, without knowing it possibly, without claiming it, she stands up for all women." - Maya Angelou

I believe in the person I have become but it didn't happen overnight. I slowly learned through life's many twists and turns that we all have a purpose and a place in this amazing world.

Regardless of who you are or what you have, girls and women everywhere share the common struggle with body images and self-esteem. I was no different.

I grew up very proud of my roots and the values instilled in me by my grandparents and aunts and uncles. They taught me both the beauty and the hardships that come along as we go about living our lives day to day, valuable lessons that I brought with me while growing up in Montreal, Canada. Throughout high school and college, I was an avid athlete, but competitive bodybuilding was not something I saw as my chosen path. I just wanted to be active.

But then life happens. For whatever reason, we take on new duties, work gets in the way, family responsibilities take over, and before we know it, the type of activeness we once knew has begun to change. Things in my life seemed to be going pretty well. I had just started my own software company after years of non-stop travelling on the road as an IT consultant. However, along with all that, I also began to notice that all I seemed to do was work and that when I wasn't working, I was too tired to do anything else.

One day, I was introduced to a friend of a friend who happened to be a professional female bodybuilder. At first all I could do was stare. As we all sat around chatting, I began to realize I was the only one asking more and more questions about how she got to her current level. The first thing she told me was that it took a lot of hard work, discipline, and commitment, which was something I had never shied away from.

I didn't start out to become a competitive bodybuilder. Like so many others, before me, it was about getting healthy and fit. And like everything else in my life, whenever I want to do something or achieve something, I visualize what my end goal is. I would then set small milestones that would help me to reach the bigger ones, and I would celebrate each and every success. If I had down times, then I had down times, and I never berated myself when I did. The mind can be a very powerful friend or your own worst foe. It listens to everything you tell it.

And I listened very carefully, to everyone around me but more importantly to myself and what my body would tell me was possible and what was not. I never forced myself to do what others were doing but instead focused on my own goals and what I wanted for myself. Just like that female bodybuilder said, it does take hard work and commitment. But I just kept setting those milestones and each one just became another challenge, another bar that I wanted to reach.

Within my first year of competing, I reached national status. Four years later, I went on to win the coveted IFBB Pro Card and became a Professional Athlete. I feel very blessed whenever I see my picture or an article about me in a sports magazine. I am thrilled to have achieved such a status in professional sports while never losing sight of the journey to get here.

Along all my different paths, though, I had never thought of myself as a role model. Not because I didn't believe in my own gifts or questioned whether I had any: I just didn't think of leadership. That is, until the day one of my best friends came to me in tears asking for my help. When she told me that she wanted to be like me, I just stared at her, somewhat confused, waiting for her to make one of her usual teasing comments. She had heard me talk about fitness and nutrition and living a healthy lifestyle for years, and in all that time, she would tease me endlessly about my somewhat casual chats on nutrition and meal preparation. More than once I tried to explain to her that what goes into your body matters, but she would walk off laughing and commenting about how obsessed I was and how that was "so not her."

Standing in my living room that day, Sue wasn't laughing. After battling health issues for many years, she realized that regular gym visits were not in the cards for her. Frustrated and growing despondent, she blurted out, "I just feel so heavy, even walking up the stairs. And look at my stomach. It's growing!" As with most women, when we gain weight, we tend to gain it around our mid-section, and this was becoming a growing concern for Sue. She often felt out of breath and fatigued and kept up a long running commentary about how her clothes were shrinking on a regular basis, to which I would just nod and smile as friends would sometimes do.

But this time, her heartfelt cry for help was something I could not ignore. "You have to listen to what I tell you and follow through on it," was the first thing I said.

I had never seen her so fired up in all the years I've known her. "I promise. You teach me, show me what to do and I will do it," she said. "I'm tired of feeling like this. Not to mention, I want to look good in a t-shirt, one that doesn't feel like it's strangling me. I know that might seem petty, but it's just something simple for me."

On a daily basis over the next few months, Sue and I talked about nutrition and fitness. Her health issues limited the activities available to her, so walking became her rep of choice. Sue's biggest change was in her relationship to food. She was an emotional eater. If she got upset, it was often off to McDonald's to ease the pain. If she was feeling sick, out came the Pringles. I shared with her what I had learned on my journey to a healthier lifestyle. I showed her how to make protein shakes, which she took on more than enthusiastically, and how to balance her meals with respect to proteins and carbs. One of her favorite morning meals was comprised of half a cup of oatmeal mixed with water and heated in the microwave, topped and blended with berries and a scoop of whey protein powder. As she got more comfortable, I would see her adding stevia, flaxseed oil, and cinnamon. There was no stopping her.

Even though Sue had mentioned to me many times in the past that she wanted to lose weight and have a healthier lifestyle, I never saw her more focused or determined than she was now. I knew she was going to tackle this head-on because it was her own decision to do so. She had been the one to come to me, and doing so seemed to give her this stronger sense of purpose. You cannot repeat the same habits, especially the not-so-good ones, every day and expect a different result. Luckily, the universe tends to let you know when you are on track and when you are off. You just get a feeling, and you know what it is. But sometimes we tend to put on blinders, especially when it involves things that we say we want to do but don't actually do. I have been guilty of that on more than one occasion.

Sue had no blinders on this time. She took ownership of what she wasn't doing and when she didn't know the exact path to take, she asked me for help. She came to me weighing in at over one hundred and fifty-five pounds, which was somewhat overweight for her height and body type. For years she had ridden that roller coaster of lose five and gain ten because because she never really changed her routine or her bad habits. Now she realized this. We also weren't on a clock, no sense of "you have to do this in this amount of time." We monitored her weight so I could know if we needed to add more protein or "good foods," but we were never chasing a number. Within her first year, Sue started to maintain a steady weight of between one hundred and twenty-seven and one hundred and thirty pounds.

It has been two years since Sue and I had that conversation in my living room, and every time I see her walking around in her baggy t-shirts, I just smile. To know that what I had taken as just a regular part of my day could be a guiding path for someone else has been one of the most humbling experiences of my life. When I look back and see all the people who helped me, it just makes sense to see the circle completes itself. When you give, you truly do receive — in so many amazing ways.

We all have personal goals that we strive to achieve. One of mine was to become a professional athlete in a sport that I am very passionate about. Yes, for me, that sport was competitive bodybuilding; this may not be the case for everyone, nor does it have to be. You get to choose your path. My journey has taught me many things but what stands out the most is that in spite of adversity and often harsh judgement, I got to choose what was right for me. And I still get to choose. I still set small milestones to reach my bigger ones, whether it is in my work life or my personal fitness goals.

I am humbled and grateful for what I have achieved over the years, both on my own and with the help and guidance of so many others who took time to teach me when I asked. Life truly is what you make it and what you put into it. In those moments when you may feel lost or unsure, remind yourself that you don't have to do everything alone. We all need help at times, a little guidance here and there. So just ask because you deserve to reap the rewards of a life well lived.

19

THE PATH TO PRIORITY: YOU!

"We only have time for the things we make a priority."

BY: JULIA LEFAIVRE

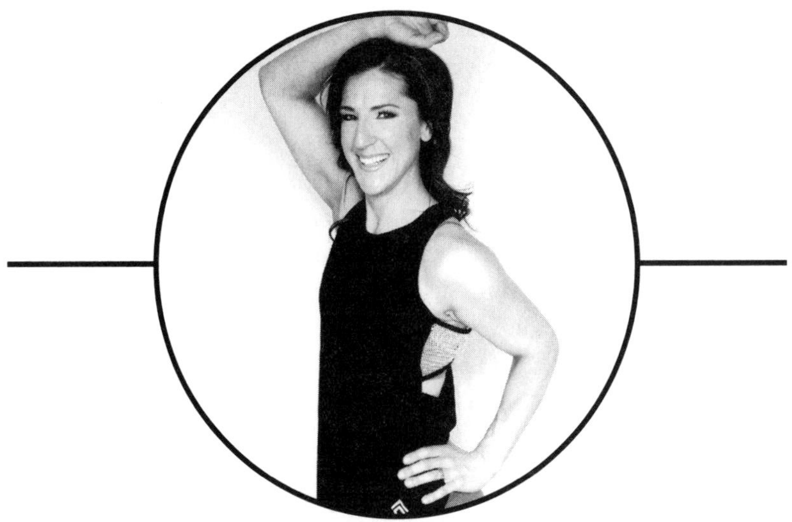

Julia Lefaivre grew up playing sports, including competitive soccer, and rowed on her university crew team. After university, though, Julia followed a different career path and became a teacher for almost ten years. When she became a mom for the first time in 2011, she found herself in lost in this new identity. She returned to teaching after both her first and her second child, but she continued to struggle with who she really was. Julia continued to be drawn back to her roots as an athlete and her love for fitness. Five years ago, while still teaching and raising her two kids, she began her online fitness business in the hopes of one day transitioning out of teaching and into the fitness industry full-time. She accomplished that dream. Not only does Julia coach women in fitness and nutrition, she also inspires women through her podcast, The Thriving Woman, and through her success coaching. This jack-of-all-trades, no-excuse momma of three works to inspire and empower women to take control of their health, regain their energy, and build strength and confidence so they can conquer any challenge life throws their way and become the best version of themselves.

I still remember those long, beautiful summer days of childhood — the warmth of the sun as it set, the sweat on my brow, and the feeling of pure bliss and joy as I spent the entire day outside, free of any care in the world. Every year my dad would plant a garden in our back field, and it seemed that year after year, the garden would get bigger and bigger. There were always new vegetables. Some years he even added new features, like archways for the beanstalks to grow on or tire stacks for potatoes. One of my favorite things to do was run to the garden for a snack: the ultimate fast food. My four siblings and I would pull a carrot straight out of the ground, hose it off with water, and dig our teeth into it. The taste of freshly picked veggies was nothing like store-bought. As I look back now, I see that my childhood garden had a huge impact on my love for food and nutrition. But healthy food was something I took for granted and didn't always prioritize in my life.

I grew up in a household where health was emphasized. Our parents encouraged us to play many sports and eat homecooked meals. That being said, we are of Polish and Italian descent, which means that even though most of our meals were homecooked, they may not have always been the healthiest or at least not the most sensible portions.

Health and fitness have always been part of my life; growing up as an athlete playing various sports, these things became a part of who I was. However, during seasons of my life, these things weren't as high on the list. More important things — studying in university, working multiple part-time jobs, partying with friends — sometimes took priority over my health. But here's the thing: we are not part of our priority list. The only option is to take care of ourselves so that we are at our best to tackle our list of priorities.

What does that mean?

It means that our health and well-being shouldn't just be a checkmark on a checklist. We can't just think that if we have time to get to it, we will and if not, we'll worry about our health tomorrow. We're not guaranteed tomorrow.

We don't belong on our priority list because we are the list. Without ourselves, no list would exist. We can't tackle our list — kids, career, spouse, friends, or housework — if we are not at our best.

When we understand the true impact and power that self-care, particularly fitness and nutrition, has over our mind, energy, and productivity, that self-care will become number one. We need to be the best in our health so we have the best of ourselves to give to those around us.

As a woman, wife, mom of three, and business owner, I know quite well how important it is to be my healthiest version. When I take care of myself, I am more creative and focused in my business. I am more present and calmer as a mom. I am more vibrant and have an increased sex drive for my spouse, and I am stronger and more confident as a woman. Our health needs to be at the top of our list. We need to fill our cup first.

I recently listened to a TEDtalk about the short-term and long-term benefits of exercise. Importantly, exercise brings us focus. "[A] single workout can improve your ability to shift and focus attention and that focus improvement will last for at least two hours."[1]

The truth is, we have the ability to get things done. We can be more productive to tackle our priority list. Take a look at the women you know who seem to be crushing it. Yes, they struggle, too; their lives are not perfect. But instead of being jealous, look at what they are doing. I'd bet they are taking time for themselves and prioritizing their health. Use them as an example of what is possible for our lives, health, and happiness.

When it comes to fitness, I have done it all. Okay, not quite everything: I have yet to try CrossFit, but that is on my goal list for this year. I have played individual sports and team sports, done rowing and running, completed triathlons, and even competed in a couple of fitness competitions. Through it all, each sport, coach, and early morning training taught me lessons of growth, determination, teamwork, and strength. I have carried these lessons with me throughout my life and transferred them into my career as a leader and success coach.

My body and my fitness mission have transformed over the years, but one thing remains constant: my health is a priority. Especially now, more than ever, as a mom of three and a multi-business owner. We don't have a nanny or support or help from family

[1] Suzuki, Wendy. (2017, November). Wendy Suzuki: The brain-changing benefits of exercise [Video file]. Retrieved from https://www.ted.com/talks/wendy_suzuki_the_brain_changing_benefits_of_exercise?language=e n

(although I'm sure they would help if we didn't live on the other side of the country), but I still prioritize myself. If something is important to us, we need to make time for it; otherwise it doesn't happen. It's not just about health; this also relates to everything else: date night with your spouse, time with friends, or your business. If it's important enough to us, we'll make time; if not, we'll make an excuse.

I didn't always have this fact figured out. In fact, I really used to take my health for granted. I didn't know what fit was and honestly, I never really noticed my body. Maybe that's a good thing. As I mentioned earlier, I grew up in a small house in the country, spending lots of time outdoors. We ate healthy, homecooked meals and in the summer a lot of our food came from the garden. Our nutrition wasn't perfect, but I didn't ever worry about what I ate. I loved the food and I ate a lot, and I mean *a lot,* of food. As an athlete, I had a revving metabolism. I really could eat whatever I wanted without visible consequence. Lucky me, right?!

Well, not so much. The consequences of not truly understanding nutrition and the impact it had on overall health, not just on weight, hit me when I began a new lifestyle as a university student. The combination of my new, more sedentary lifestyle, paired with the mindset that I could eat whatever I wanted, resulted in a weight gain of thirty pounds over three years, as well as numerous health problems. I was tired all the time, my iron levels were so low they were almost undetectable, and my energy level was low. I remember hanging out with my cousins the summer after my second year of university. I felt uncomfortable in my clothes and kept pulling at my shirt. Everything was too tight. I went to lie on the hammock with two family members when I heard someone calling from across the yard, "Ummm, that really isn't made for more than two people." It was a large hammock. Earlier that day, there had been multiple people on it. This was the first time I really became self-conscious of my body. I felt uncomfortable and ashamed.

Something needed to change. I was still active but my nutrition was lacking. I ate healthy when I could, but on a student budget, I could only afford pasta and a few fruits and veggies. The lifestyle was slowly killing me, not just physically but emotionally as well. Then I took a class on behavior modification in my last semester of university.

This class began the change for me, helping me learn how to set a goal and create an action plan to achieve it.

To start my plan, I had to figure out what life after "athlete" looked like, what fitness would look like for me in the future. In order to be healthy, we have to align our goal with healthy actions, *daily*. I enrolled in a running class at the local Running Room. Each week we would begin with a lesson on stretching, breathing, running, and even nutrition. I really enjoyed being a part of a community again; it's what I had loved about being an athlete on a team and what I had missed. Within three months, I had lost ten pounds; three months after that, I lost the next ten.

I had started to feel like myself again, strong like an athlete, but I still wasn't feeling my best. I knew something more needed to change. I still carried the mentality that I could eat what I wanted to a certain extent. As long as I didn't overeat, I thought I could outwork my bad nutrition choices.

Wrong!

My now-husband and I began training for a mini-ultramarathon (twenty-five kilometers), but I just didn't feel like a runner. I wasn't lean like I thought a runner should be, and always felt heavy on my feet, even though I was twenty pounds lighter than on the day I took my very first running class. We decided to try P90X, an at-home workout program, although we were skeptical. My goal was not to lose weight but to get toned and lean. After ninety days of following the fitness program and of following a structured nutrition plan for the first time ever, I gained muscles, became lean and toned, and lost the last ten pounds. I was blown away.

My experience with P90X opened my eyes to an entirely new fitness world: strength training and nutrition. All these years, I had eaten healthy but struggled with really understanding what to eat, how much to eat, and when to eat it. Things didn't really change until I did the research and paired a great fitness routine with a *proper*, certified nutrition program. *Boom!* Who knew? That is where the magic happened. It really was that simple.

Here's the thing: through all the different seasons of my life, from struggling with my weight in university to rediscovering what fitness looked like as an adult, health has always been a part of my identity. Fitness is not just a size or a look; it's a feeling: strength, confidence, *energy*. Have I mentioned I have three young kids? I need all the energy I can get!

Now that I am grown with children of my own, I find myself drawn back to the days of picking fresh veggies from my dad's garden. I teach my kids to have the same love for fresh food by planting our own garden each summer; just like my dad's, it gets bigger and bigger every year.

Over a lifetime of ups and downs with my own health journey, I have learned what works and that is to keep it simple: move more and nourish my body with whole foods. I have been blessed to have had health and fitness as part of my life; they has taught me so many lessons. My passion for nutrition and health doesn't just stop with my family's dinner table, either. It has grown into a desire to empower other women and families to shoot higher when it comes to prioritizing their health and taking the time to learn about food and nutrition. After a ten-year teaching career, I was inspired to take that passion and pay it forward, and I left my career as a teacher. For last five years, I have been empowering women to start their own health journey and become their own health leaders and advocates. I teach women to do their research, try new foods, and track what they eat to see what works for their body. Some foods are natural and healthy but your body may not digest them well. We just need to pay attention. Over the last year I have evolved as leader and in my business. I became certified to coach people through the customization of a health and nutrition plan to their lifestyle and goals. As well as taking it further to not just coach women in health and fitness. I do group and one-on-one coaching for women in all areas of their life. Teaching them to be unapologetic about their goals, dream big and to create clear action plans and success habits so that they can live life to their full potential. My goal is to help women feel strong, confident, and energized in both their health, life, relationships and career/business. It's time, ladies, to make your goals a priority!

20

EMPOWER THE WORLD WITH YOUR PRESENCE

*"Take your place. Step into your power.
Share love with the world through your presence."*

BY: LOLA T. SMALL

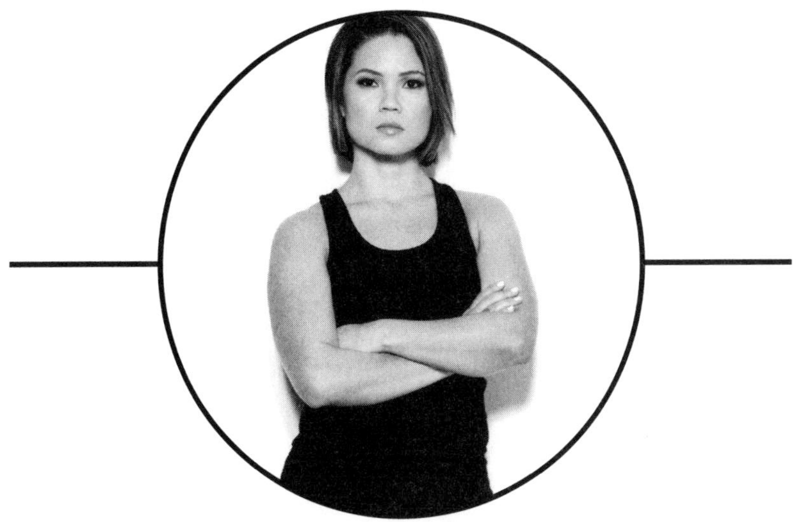

Lola T. Small is a growth and success coach for emerging women healers, leaders, and change-makers. Through body-mind-life empowerment teaching and events, Lola inspires and guides women around the world to build true strength within and to share their best selves with the world. She grew up with two sisters in Asia, where the culture favors boys, and is passionate about uplifting girls and women to their highest potential and empowering women to share their talents and dreams for positive social change.

Having split her time between the East and the West and having lived without her family since the age of fifteen, Lola has had to go through many layers of self-discovery to define who she truly is. Extensive inner work in her twenties has given Lola a tremendous sense of self, clarity about her passions and purpose, and a tenacious drive to share her positively powerful energy and love around the globe.

A lover of heartfelt connections, world travel to beautiful oceans, strength training, and destination half marathons, Lola loves her fun life with her husband, Shawn, and son Jordie.

www.lolasmall.com

fb: @lolatsmall | ig: @lolatsmall

RISE AND THRIVE

The other day, a friend vented to me about how frustrated she was, feeling stuck between taking care of her two-year-old son amid toddler tantrums and wanting time for herself to pursue her dreams. I hear it all too often: tired mamas who say over and over how much they would like to lose weight and be fit, only to jump from fad diets to not doing anything at all, feeling stagnant and defeated.

We are here for a special reason, and we owe it to ourselves and to our loved ones to find out what that is. But being a mother, wife, and all the other roles we women play in life is demanding enough; forget about figuring who we are, how to make our dreams come true, and how to feel fit and fabulous in our bodies. So many of us live in basic survival mode, so how do we make our way to optimal wellness and our best life? Where do we start? How is it even possible when it feels like we have to take care of the whole world?

As an empowerment coach and trainer for women, and a mom myself, I am passionate about helping women rise above the frustrations and move toward fulfillment. It is my mission every day to remind women that yes, we are here to do something impactful with our lives, especially if we have little eyes watching. We are here to share our energy and our presence with the world, so let's rise and thrive. Let me share with you how our fitness journeys can help us get there.

THE SECRET SAUCE

As a young girl growing up in Asia, I was taught to be "ladylike": demure and obedient. I was encouraged to follow the rules set out for women, which means finding a good husband, having babies, and living happily ever after. Luckily for me, my father wanted a different future for us, so he moved our family to the U.S. when I was eleven and I got to have experiences that allowed me to see a different reality.

After tennis practice one day during my senior year in high school, a friend asked me to spot him in the weight room. I didn't know it, but this experience would change me for life. The raw power, incredible energy, and rush of endorphins — I had gotten my first taste of how powerful my body could be. I fell in love with strength training, and it has been an anchor in my life ever since. A few years later, and ironically back in Asia, I stepped into the world of fitness. I began to teach spinning, yoga, and circuit training, and I loved every sweaty minute!

My journey led me back to North America where I pursued my passion in personal growth and empowerment work. After several years of full-time jobs, part-time coaching, marriage, and kids, I am now happily home in my heart as I support other women on their journeys to strength, power, and potential. For all my women, especially mommies, who are yearning for a little bit more of yourself, wondering how you can rise above it all and own your power, I share with you my secret sauce.

1. INVEST IN SELF-DISCOVERY.

Honor yourself and your journey; take the time to find your individuality instead of blindly following what is expected of you from family and society. Dedicating time and effort to my personal growth has resulted in some of the richest experiences I have created for myself. I know my strengths, weaknesses, values, purpose, passions, and dreams. Knowing myself well allows me to be strong in my convictions in daily life, from what I say to how I act to what to say yes or no to when life offers unlimited choices and opportunities. Sometimes we may feel guilty or selfish for taking time to focus on us, but the deep inner knowing that we gain when we know the core of who we are serves a much greater purpose.

The more I knew myself, the more I liked who I was and started to truly enjoy spending time with my own being. I learned to love myself instead of seeking approval from others, and I became comfortable in my skin. I love reading personal growth books, learning from others by going to workshops and retreats, and taking quiet time to reflect and journal, even if it's only for five minutes each day.

We are our closest companions for the rest of our lives. Let's truly get to know ourselves well.

2. KNOW WHAT YOU WANT IN LIFE.

In addition to learning who we are, getting clear on our passions and purpose brings so much power to how we live our everyday lives. I love asking myself, "What do I love, what do I want to achieve and experience in this lifetime, and how do I want to make a difference by being here?" These are profound and such life-changing questions, ones that only we and our own souls know how to answer.

My life became impactful and meaningful when I defined what I wanted it to be about. When I gained clarity about how I wanted to create my life, I discovered newfound focus and drive. I started sharing my passions, creating fun and memorable experiences, checking things off my bucket list, and giving back to my communities. I now look for opportunities to share my life purpose in everything I do, and life is full of ease, flow, and love.

Have fun identifying what means the most to you so that you can design a life you love. My motto has always been, "We have one life to live, so let's make it the most amazing one we can!"

3. LEARN TO TURN DREAMS INTO ACTIONS.

Perhaps the biggest thing that fitness has taught me is the practice and discipline of taking action. Oh yes, there have been countless times when I didn't feel up to working out or felt too tired to care about my goals. But over and over, I go back to the weights and crank out the reps, even if it's only three exercises in my pajamas in my basement home gym! The repeated act of showing up is the way we make things happen. We achieve our fitness and wellness goals when we work out and eat healthy foods on a consistent basis. Likewise, we meet our personal and life dreams when we take daily action in alignment with our vision and intention.

Life doesn't care whether we take tiny actions or massive actions; it just asks us to keep the forward momentum alive by doing. Stay in motion with the things we say are important to us, and life will do its share to propel us along. On those days when I've had a rough night because my toddler didn't want to sleep or when piles of laundry have been sitting around for a week, I give myself room for compassion and rest when I need. But when the energy comes back and I remind myself of my vision, I start again and take action to keep moving forward until my goals and dreams are fulfilled.

It feels truly affirming and empowering when we see the fruits of our labor. Our dedication, patience, and perseverance while we do the work will lead us to the strong physique, beautiful health, and dream life we desire.

4. BUILD A CONFIDENT AND POSITIVE PRESENCE.

When I go into the gym and see all the people lifting the weights and pounding along on the treadmill, I often wonder what they're thinking in their heads. Maybe they're thinking about what to make for dinner, about bills and money, or about how much longer they need to be on this thing. I have come to really cherish my training times, especially when I lift and run, because I have turned it into a time when I focus my thoughts on what I want to create and manifest. My time to move my body in connection with my breath is also my "power up" time for my mind.

Let me teach you how to get the biggest bang for your buck whenever you move and sweat.

Whatever goal or dream I am pursuing at the moment, I use my workout time to focus my mind on seeing myself succeeding at those goals. I pick one or two powerful affirmations and repeat them in my head as I rep out those deadlifts. When I put in those kilometers for half marathon training, I forgo the music, and direct my focus on feeling myself celebrating a dream come true. Imagining being on cloud nine makes my runs feel amazing and literally takes me one step closer to those dreams!

The energy from this repeated practice of feeling positive, strong, powerful, and confident while moving my body carries over to my everyday life. It makes me feel optimistic, radiant, and successful. I enjoy and look forward to my workouts because I know I will leave empowered and exuding the most powerful after-glow. Our fitness practice gives us the opportunity to cultivate true inner confidence that radiates happy vibes on the outside. Don't go through another workout without flexing this new visualization muscle!

5. SHARE OURSELVES WITH POWER AND LOVE.

I feel a deep sense of responsibility to teach other women what I've learned and to help them see fitness in a different way and use it as a tool for personal empowerment and life manifestation. Whether it's with my family, my friends, or my coaching and training clients, I have the power to encourage a new way of thinking about how we move our bodies and how we focus our minds when we move. When we discover our own power, we then have the privilege of sharing that power with someone else so that they may know theirs. What an extraordinary way to turn something as ordinary as working out into a phenomenal tool of imparting power and love to another person.

I use what I have learned from my time in the weight room to teach others to bring out the power within themselves. My journey to bring out my mental best as I work on my physical best has allowed me to see that people who struggle with weight or fitness are all just looking for the same things: self-belief, self-affirmation, and a sense of power and love. When we are open, we can start to give ourselves and others all these things we crave from a deep place in our beings.

How can we share ourselves and our power? We can invite someone to join us for a workout so they can enjoy the many benefits of exercise and social time. We can get to know what type of activity our partner enjoys and spend quality and healthy time together. We can teach our children to learn patience, persistence, hard work, and dedication by practicing and mastering a sport. We can notice and give a sincere compliment when we see another woman making great efforts to take care of herself instead of commenting on superficial things like weight loss. And we can lend a hand and show someone else the ropes at the gym, helping them feel comfortable and empowered.

POWER UP FOR LIFE

There was a time in my twenties when I taught fitness and yoga full time. During this period, I aspired to be as fit as the models you see on the cover of fitness magazines and in fitness competitions. I counted how much protein I ate, I stressed hard in the grocery store over which cookies would do the least amount of damage to my hard-earned physique, and I even made myself throw up those cookies after binging an entire box one night. My love for fitness had gone too far, past what felt good and right, and I had to take a step back to re-evaluate what I was doing to myself. Being obsessed to the point of disordered eating was unhealthy for my body and destructive for my mind and spirit. I am grateful I had the awareness and the opportunity to shift and make a change.

Almost two decades later when I had our first baby at age thirty-eight, I finally recognized my body's true power and gave it the real love it deserves. My perspective on fitness and working out has transformed as my gratitude for my body has taken front and center. What once used to be a pursuit born out of not feeling good enough is now a privilege and a joy that adds power and energy to my everyday life. I no longer count how many egg whites I'm eating, beat myself up for not getting six workout sessions in for the week, or obsess about how my tummy has this slight roll if I lower my pants a certain way. I now focus on the power I feel when I lift, on the energy I get from my runs, and on how much our son loves copying my squat presses with his own set of one-pound dumbbells.

Our physical practice and bodywork can serve as a tool that empowers our lives in the direction we want it to go. From the way we see ourselves to how we feel about who we are and how we are here to affect the world, our fitness journey can sharpen our mental focus, increase our happiness and well-being, and deepen our love for ourselves and those around us.

We have been given the gift of a body that is capable of running, lifting, stretching, and playing. Our gift back to life is to fully use that body to own our power in being here. Let's take our place, power up, and use our phenomenal energy to inspire, uplift, and make an impact with our time on earth.

21

FREE TO BE ME

"It is not the circumstances in life that define us but rather how we choose to make every situation a means to better ourselves and the lives around us."

BY: DEIRDRE SLATTERY

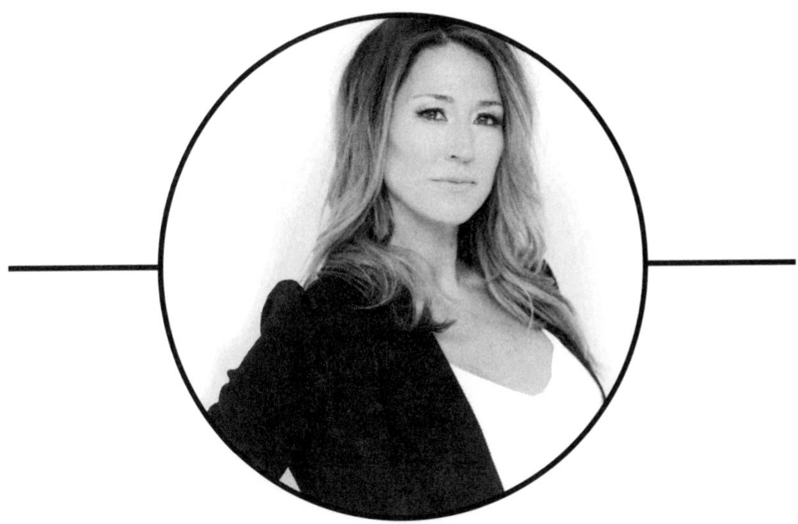

Deirdre Slattery is a single mother of a beautiful daughter who is the greatest support and has brought out Deirdre's passion to live her best: healthy, positive, and as a strong, independent woman. She sees change as a constant opportunity to learn and grow and to make the best of life around her. Deidre is an eternal optimist with a grounded and practical balance. Helping others to see their potential comes naturally to her, and finding the good in every situation makes her life work meaningful. Deidre's purpose is to inspire and motivate others to stay positive and strong in the face of any adversity.

This free spirit has traveled the globe learning about life and feels especially at home near the ocean with people who are healthy, thriving, and happy. Deidre received a bachelor's of kinesiology and education from the University of Windsor, where she majored in biology and health education. After twenty years, she is following her heart and expanding her career to educate and coach others to live healthy and happy lives. Nutrition, exercise, and a healthy mindset make up the foundations of her healthy lifestyle, and her future plans as an entrepreneur include making a greater impact in the health and fitness industry and lifestyle coaching. Deirdre finds the most reward in helping others unlock and overcome their barriers a life they dream of. She is open-minded and open-hearted and there to listen and guide others to live their best in health and wellness.

www.deirdreslattery.arbonne.com

ig: @deirdre_sfitness

Somewhere along my career path, I started longing and searching for more out of life. I would dream of different jobs and things I wanted to cross off my bucket list, only to talk myself out of those dreams. *It's too late, you could never do that.* That little voice convinced me to continue doing what I knew day in and day out, year after year, leaving me feeling discontent and longing for more out of life. While ignoring my heart's desires and playing it safe kept me stable for many years — think job security, pension and health benefits —I felt like I was short-changing myself, not living up to my potential.

Sometimes it seems easier to stay small and safe than to live the life you are dreaming of by owning and acting on your big, scary goals. But we only have this one life to live. I know I want to make the best life I can by taking steps past my fears and toward my dreams. No matter how hard it is, that's more satisfying and rewarding than living with what-ifs and regret.

The turning point in my life came four months before my forty-fourth birthday. I had been dreading my birthday every year since I turned thirty-nine. Forty was an especially trying year for me: an early mid-life crisis, you might call it. I was not anywhere close to the life I wished to be living when it came to my career, my romantic relationship, and my financial status. While I loved my daughter, my family, and my long-standing friendships, I wanted more freedom, creativity, and autonomy in my career and more control over how I lived my life. I no longer wanted to be dependent on others to give me a sense of security, financially, personally, or professionally. I was ready to step into the woman I had only begun to dream I could be: happy in my skin and in my own company, with a healthy heart and mind that would not be impacted by others' words or actions. To be truly free, I knew I needed to cultivate a mindset of inner peace. I needed to believe that I was enough for myself and for others who were worthy and deserving of my time, energy, work, and love. My goal became to feel secure in who I am and undeterred by life circumstances. It was time to get real with myself and live my best, most authentic life: not based on societal pressures and norms, not for family or friends, but for me.

My relationship with health and fitness had always come relatively easily and naturally. I loved sports and being active, especially outdoors, and I loved to eat food that was delicious and mostly nutritious. I ate well and I stayed healthy and fit. In my thirties, though, I started to become a little more preoccupied with my health and body image. Since having a child and working full time, I didn't feel like I had time for myself to focus on being active or going to the gym. This was when my questions about life started. Was I really happy with where I was? As a single mom, I was making decisions, or more like compromises. I felt that it was time to make things "work" and to settle down to make a life — that was what we were supposed to do, right? I stayed in relationships that were far below the bar for what I wanted in a partner because of my age and my situation; I felt obligated to make them work because I introduced my daughter to these men. In reality, I was slowly adopting a lower standard for what my daughter and I needed in our lives. I was forcing things to work and trying so desperately that I was losing sight of my worth. In the end, these failed relationships, which I now can appreciate were all part of the bigger plan to help me regain my sense of self, turned out to be lessons and blessings that helped shape me and prepare me for the best yet to come.

Being single, parenting alone, and hitting forty all lay heavy in my heart and had me feeling quite low. The little cracks in my self-esteem became bigger until I was no longer complete; I started to believe I was not enough. It's a feeling I had experienced before in relationships, both friendships and romances, that weren't good for my soul. Now at forty, I started to feel the same in my workplace. I had lost myself somewhere in others' opinions, in stories I allowed to fill my heart and head about who I was. For a girl who had always believed in herself, I felt very alone and depressed about my future.

I knew I had to take control of my life and my well-being and stand up for myself. I wanted my daughter to see me rise in the face of hardship and come back to who I had always been. What I have learned about myself since that time is that there is always more in me to become.

Secretly, I had watched the lives of fitness athletes, competitors, and models in awe, wishing I could do that, too. The life I was leading at the time had me believing and accepting that it was too late and that I wasn't capable of achieving these goals. Then I met one of these icons and badass rock stars in person. Finally, I got the chance to vocalize this dream someone who would understand and say, "Hell yes, girl!"

I had watched and admired Bunny Azzopardi for years, wondering how she did it and thinking that I would love not only to look that good but to take a secret dream and make it a reality. Meeting Bunny was a perfectly timed moment. She was more than I had imagined her to be: open, honest, and real with me. Inspired, I set out to get my ass, and my life in shape within two months of meeting her.

I was four months shy of forty-four when I finally said, "Enough! It's time to make yourself accountable and shine." I went from barely being able to get outside, showered, and dressed by 3pm when my daughter got home from school to driving twice a week for an hour and a half to meet my trainer and put my goals into action. I wanted to take my health and fitness to a new level, to the uncomfortable edge and beyond to become my best. No longer would I accept living below the mark I was shooting for; now I was committed to doing all I could to reach my potential and see what was inside of me. It was on. I made a video and posted it on social media so everyone could hear me state my intention to transform my life from the inside out, starting with nutrition and fitness. I was excited and felt alive, full of purpose. My "Four to Forty-Four" journey had begun, and I gave myself a goal, a timeline, a coach, and a plan to see it happen. Over the next four months, I examined my intentions and my lifelong views on health and fitness, and I shifted them from a place of obligation to get in shape for a season to a commitment to my body, mind, and spirit. To level up and reach new heights in any area of life, we will only succeed with commitment — not a "have to" mindset but a choice to commit to the process. Once you watch the results come in, the motivation to keep going will trickle into other areas of your life.

I had started my mission to better my life, and the fall-out and the ripple effect brought me more than the best physical shape I have ever been in. The journey brought me a love and appreciation for what my healthy and able body could do once my mind was attached to and connected to the goal. The peace gained, the clarity experienced, and the after-effects of each workout brought me back day after day. During every workout, I practiced gratitude for being able to move my body and exercise my mind.

In the beginning, some workouts brought me to tears as I let go of old tapes in my head and shifted my thoughts to strong, powerful statements. I used these like a mantra to push my limits and break the barriers I had allowed to come up around me. *I am strong. I can. I am winning. I am worthy.* I repeated these statements in my mind, especially during heavier lifts and on days the cardio was tough, and they remain part of my mantras today. Fitness doesn't get easier; there isn't a magic threshold that, once crossed, makes getting the work done simpler. It will always be challenging, especially when other life factors are weighing on you. But the commitment you have made to yourself, the hours put in, the improvements you have made and felt, the connection between your mind and your body: those will keep you on track.

For me, the dedication to achieving my goal was the catalyst to making changes in my way of thinking about what I could achieve in the rest of my life. I landed on my forty-fourth birthday feeling joyful, accomplished, and lighter in my heart. Seeing my goal through and starting to see my light shining again, not for anyone else but myself, broke my pattern of feeling broken and depressed. Now I knew that can achieve more, I can dream of more, and I can want more. What else is possible?

The gym was there for me from the time I was a happy, carefree teen through my twenties, when I was loving and living out loud, and my thirties, when I was focused on getting ready to fit into my bikini on March break. In my forties, it became more than all of that. It became my freedom, my safe place, my second home, and my daily break. It showed me how much more I could do when I set my mind to it and became the space where I could elevate my life.

ACKNOWLEDGMENTS:

Thank you to my parents, Dr. Dennis and LTC Harriett Rowe, for providing me with a foundation of optimism. To Vince, Piper, Brynn, and Jordan, thank you for your encouragement and supporting me in yet another endeavor.

- Allison Marschean

A special thank you to my children who inspire me to be playful daily and remind me to stay open to new ways of doing things and grateful for the little things that makes us all different.

- Barb Sotos

None of this would have been possible without the love and support of my parents, inspiration from my amazing kids, and forgiveness from my husband, John, for pulling the bait-and-switch with the girl he married. An ultimate thank you goes to my besties, Skarch and Right Tit, for talking me through the bad days and last but not least to Deirdre Slattery and Golden Brick Road Publishing for giving me the opportunity to tell my story and hopefully help other women share theirs.

- Erica Glassford

There are so many people I am grateful for who have assisted me on my health journey and in my education to improve my practice. Thank you to my family, mentors, practitioners, friends, and teams; because of you, I am able to live my best life and assist many others to do so.

- Heather Chapman

To every girl who chases sunsets and believes in the power of her own voice. And to Dev for holding space for me to do the same.

- Jocelyn Hinz

To my husband Gerard, thank you for demonstrating what it means to stick with your commitment. To my boys, Noah and Jacob, thank you for giving me a reason to do better.

- Pauline Caballero

To Andrea Roszell, former classmate, roommate, fellow Body-Pump instructor, and forever friend. Thank you for getting me started on my group fitness instructor journey.

- Karen Swyszcz

Thank you to my parents and my sisters, Lena and Lisa, for supporting my life path even if they didn't agree with it or fully understand it. My biggest gratitude and love to my husband Shawn and son Jordie for being my rocks and my greatest loves.

- Lola T. Small

Thanks to all the women in my family before me; my mother Juleen, my sister Leslee, "Mothers", grandmother Silvia, great great grandmother Rachel. Maria Balunsat and all the Balunsats on down the lineage who pioneered with strength and vision making it possible for me to become the woman I am today in a world where I can own a business, speak on stage, be a competitive athlete, write and express myself, and ultimately grow into my full human potential. It is no small feat what women have accomplished over the past century.

- Rachel Balunsat

To my incredible man, Dan: your love and humor are embedded in my heart. To my extraordinary offspring: you three rock! To my forever friend, Susie: you are always with me.

- Johanne Walker

I would like to Thank my mother Sharon Rochard who is the strongest woman I know and to all of the strong women in this world. Rise to be them, Get to know them, Commit to raising them. A Special Thank you to my children who believe in me no matter what and GRB publishing for giving me and other women a platform to share their stories and gain confidence along the way.

- Sharlene Rochard

I would like to thank everyone who has inspired me to pursue my goals and has inspired this book to bring together strong women with a story behind their success to share and give back to others along their own fitness journey.

Thank you to each co-author for bringing their story to life to create this book full of passion, heart and vetted experience.

And a special thankyou to my daughter, Lily for always giving me reason to continue to build, to be strong and make a difference with my life and to share it with others.

- Deirdre Slattery

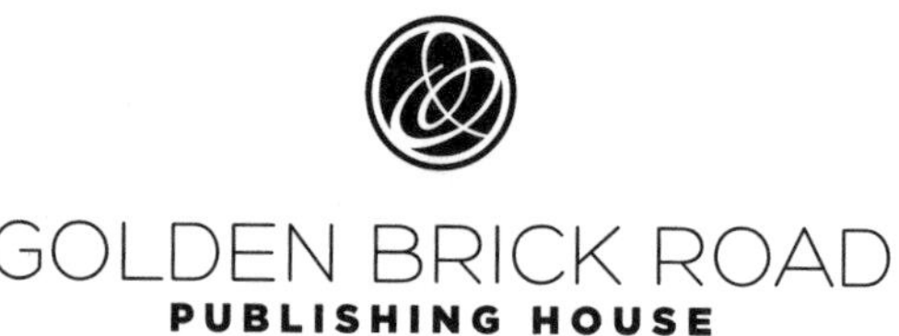

Link arms with us as we pave new paths to a better and more expansive world.

Golden Brick Road Publishing House (GBRPH) is a small, independently initiated boutique press created to provide social-innovation entrepreneurs, experts, and leaders a space in which they can develop their writing skills and content to reach existing audiences as well as new readers.

Serving an ambitious catalogue of books by individual authors, GBRPH also boasts a unique co-author program that capitalizes on the concept of "many hands make light work." GBRPH works with our authors as partners. Thanks to the value, originality, and fresh ideas we provide our readers, GBRPH books are now available in bookstores across North America.

We aim to develop content that effects positive social change while empowering and educating our members to help them strengthen themselves and the services they provide to their clients.

Iconoclastic, ambitious, and set to enable social innovation, GBRPH is helping our writers/partners make cultural change one book at a time.

Inquire today at www.goldenbrickroad.pub

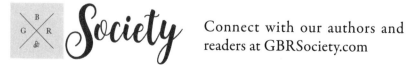

Connect with our authors and readers at GBRSociety.com